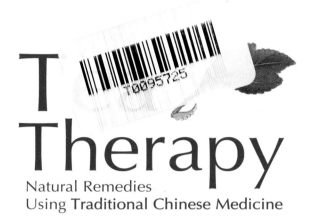

Therapy

Natural Remedies
Using **Traditional Chinese Medicine**

By Lin Qianliang & Chen Xiaoyi

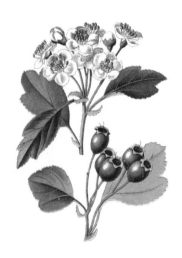

Better Link Press

Copyright © 2014 Shanghai Press and Publishing Development Co., Ltd.

Text by Lin Qianliang, Chen Xiaoyi
Translation by Cao Jianxin, Yang Lin
Photos by Liu Shenghui, Ding Guoxing, Getty Images, Quanjing
Front Cover Design by Wang Wei
Interior and Back Cover Design by Li Jing, Zhong Yiming (Yuan Yinchang
  Design Studio)

Copy Editor: Kirstin Mattson
Editor: Wu Yuezhou
Editorial Director: Zhang Yicong

ISBN: 978-1-60220-147-7

Address any comments about *Tea Therapy: Natural Remedies Using Traditional
  Chinese Medicine* to:

Shanghai Press and Publishing Development Co., Ltd.
Floor 5, No. 390 Fuzhou Road, Shanghai, China (200001)
Email: sppd@sppdbook.com

Printed in China by Shanghai Donnelley Printing Co., Ltd.

3 5 7 9 10 8 6 4

The material in this book is provided for informational purposes only and is not
intended as medical advice. The information contained in this book should not be
used to diagnose or treat any illness, disorder, disease or health problem. Always
consult your physician or health care provider before beginning any treatment of any
illness, disorder or injury. Use of this book, advice, and information contained in this
book is at the sole choice and risk of the reader.

Contents

Foreword

Tea originates from China, and time-honored, extensive and profound tea culture also stems from here. Traditional Chinese medicine (TCM) and its treatments are true Chinese national treasures. Since ancient times, tea has been closely related to TCM, which can be seen from many records on tea in classics of TCM of different dynasties. Therefore, tea is also a kind of TCM. Tea therapy is a combination of the two subjects of tea science and TCM science.

The term "tea therapy" was first proposed by Professor Lin Qianliang from Zhejiang Chinese Medical University in 1983. In 1985, he issued more than twenty articles in a special tea therapy column in a newspaper. From 1993 to 1996, he went on to present the theme of tea therapy eleven times in the journal *Tea*, as well as speaking several times at international conferences on tea culture convened in China and Japan. To date, Professor Lin Qianliang has published many relevant works in China and foreign countries, and exerted a profound influence on the field.

Originally a doctor of Western medicine in the department of surgery at the hospital of the Medical School of Zhejiang University, Professor Lin then studied TCM and became one of the first senior doctors to be familiar with both Western medicine and TCM. His works are marked by combination of the ancient and the modern as well as Western and traditional Chinese medicine.

This book, *Tea Therapy*, is divided into twelve chapters. Building on the general remarks of "On Tea" and "Tea Therapy," it then elaborates on theories and practices related to tea therapy incorporating clinical practice. This book makes for practical reading with rich content,

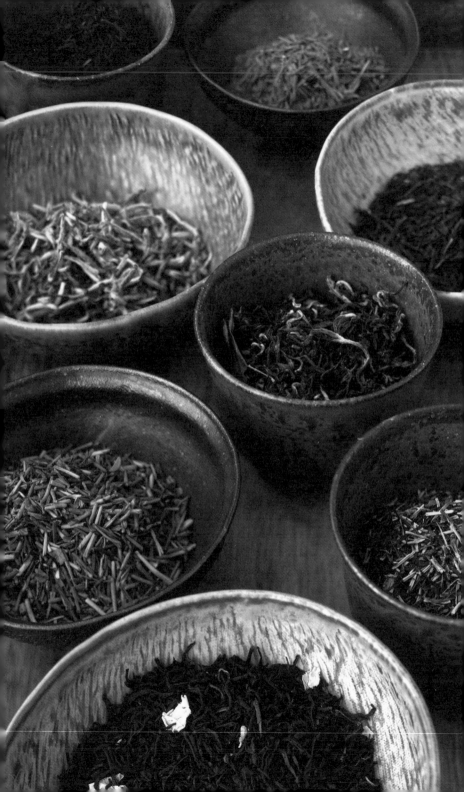

explaining profound theories in simple language. Therefore, I am pleased to recommend this book to all of you.

Liu Zusheng

(Professor Liu Zusheng, Doctoral Supervisor, is the former Dean of the Department of Tea Science, Zhejiang University, and Deputy Board Chairman of China Tea Science Society. He now serves as Senior Consultant at China's International Tea Cultural Institute.)

| Tea is a natural way for us to stay healthy.

Preface

I believe there is nothing other than the tea leaf that is so small but has such important and wide-ranging effects.

Over sixty years ago, I traveled hundreds of miles to study at the Medical School of Zhejiang University. After graduating with a bachelor's degree I stayed at the school to teach for a year, and then studied for three years at the tutorial class of traditional Chinese medicine under the jurisdiction of the Ministry of Public Health. I then conducted extensive research into the combination of Western medicine and TCM and gained some achievements.

It was around the end of the 1970s when I realized that tea was vital to many fields, such as TCM clinical practice, health-preservation, diet therapy and pharmacology, and was a major presence in materia medica. Deeply intrigued, I embarked on in-depth study of tea.

A breakthrough came in 1983 at the Cultural Symposium on Tea and Health, where two theses entitled "History of Tea" and "Effects of Tea" shocked the circle of tea science. During the discussion, I proposed the idea of "tea therapy," a system to which I have devoted the last thirty years, having now published extensively on the subject.

I reviewed about 500 sources on the effects of tea in TCM and pharmacology, having sorted out and categorized them into 24 groups. In reviewing research on the effects of tea from the perspective of "modern" medicine, I have identified twenty groups. Of course, there is a small overlap of the two categories. For example, in oral health care, both TCM and modern medicine can focus on prevention but take different approaches.

My system of tea therapy can be categorized into three groups. The

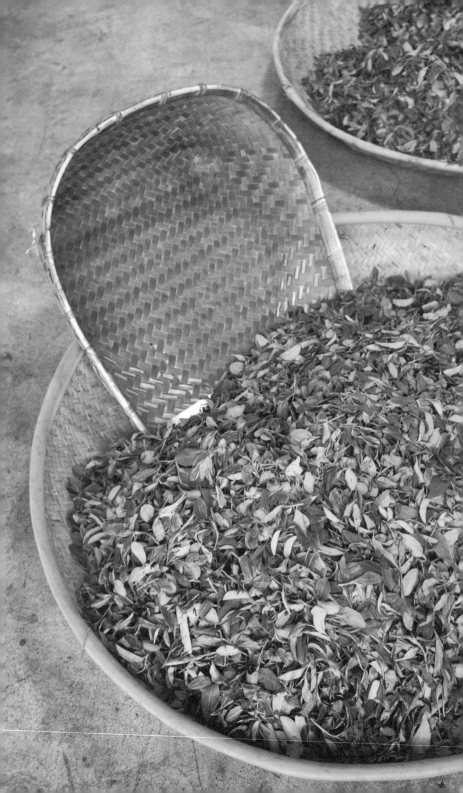

first is "single tea," which is the most basic and important group. The second is "tea and medicine" in which tea is taken together with other ingredients to enhance or modify effects. In the third, "tea substitute," tea leaves are not used but the style of drinking tea is borrowed. There is a strong tradition of drinking tea substitutes in China, as shown by the fact that dried chrysanthemum petals and rose petals are also sold in tea shops.

I have found six overall benefits of tea therapy: extensive effect, reliability of treatment and prevention, non-toxic quality, appealing taste, low price and ease of application. Even though we call it "tea therapy," more importance lies in prevention. This is in accordance with TCM, where the emphasis is placed on understanding and treating root causes of illness rather than just remedying symptoms, and taking a highly individualized approach based on the specific patient.

The tea therapies in this book help to prevent and relieve illness and pain. From the standpoint of recuperating the body, curative effects differ from person to person. To cure a disease once and for all, a doctor's advice is recommended.

"Those who drink tea can often live a longer life" is a longstanding belief in China. In fact, a common phrase, "tea-related longevity," is used to mean the age of 108. So raise a cup of tea for a long, healthy life!

Lin Qianliang

| The process of processing tea.

How to Use This Book

This book will help you prevent and treat a wide range of illnesses using time-honored, natural methods. Tea therapy is inextricably tied to traditional Chinese medicine, so it is useful to understand some basic concepts of TCM in order to use this book most effectively. And it is important to keep in mind that for severe or longstanding conditions, it is recommended that you consult with medical professionals, both of Western and traditional Chinese medicine, about your treatment.

The practice of traditional Chinese medicine, which dates back thousands of years, has grown up around several key principles such as *yin-yang, qi* and body constitution. The following provides a brief introduction; there are many books, including by this publisher, on the subject should you want to more fully explore TCM.

1. *Yin* and *yang*

This ancient concept states that there are two fundamental principles or forces in the universe, ever opposing and supplementing each other. Everything in the natural world contains two opposite components, for example, heaven and earth, outside and inside, heat and cold, etc. If *yin-yang* imbalances are found during TCM diagnosis, treatment focuses on restoring equilibrium. Of particular importance is kidney *yin* and *yang*, as kidney *yin* serves to nourish and moisten all inner organs, while kidney *yang* serves to warm and enhance all inner organs.

2. *Qi*

This refers to the vital energy, or life force, of the human body. It is the most basic substance, and it maintains activities of human life.

Qi is both the concrete substance on which the human body relies for survival and the general term for the functional activities of human organs. TCM treatment focuses on maintaining the appropriate flow of *qi* in the body.

3. Constitution

Constitution refers to the overall physical, mental and spiritual state of the body, based on the relative strength of *yin-yang* energies and different movements of *qi* and blood in the body. It is influenced both by congenital and acquired factors. Since TCM treatment is highly individualized it is important to understand your own constitution in order to select the proper course of care.

4. Body fluid

As the general term of all kinds of normal liquid in the human body, it includes body fluid contained within various human organs as well as secretions such as gastric juice, nasal mucus and tears.

5. Essence

It refers to the material basis of the human body, which maintains activities of human life, as well the basis for the growth and development of the body and for physiological and functional activities of various human organs.

6. The five organs and three visceral cavities

The five organs are the heart, liver, spleen, lungs and kidneys. They are the center for production and changes of all things resulting from *yin* and *yang*, and for storing essence and *qi*. Defined differently than in Western medicine, they include both the organ and its functional system, linked via meridians along which *qi* can flow. For example, the liver system includes not only the liver but also the gall bladder, tendons and eyes. *Jiao*, which is a noun unique to TCM, divides the body into three visceral cavities. Upper *jiao* comprises the organs above the diaphragm, middle *jiao* from below the diaphragm to the navel, and lower *jiao* below the navel.

7. Four kinds of nature

Also called the four kinds of *qi*, or temperature, in TCM, these are cool, cold, warm and hot (in addition to neutral). This relates to the relative proportion of *yin* and *yang*, and is an inherent property not necessarily dependant on surface temperature. It is important to understand your own nature as well as the nature of the food or medicine you take. For example, food or medicine of a cool or cold nature (*yin*) suits people with a hot constitution or disease (too much *yang* or deficient *yin*).

8. The five tastes

In TCM each food or herb has a certain "taste," e.g., sweet, bitter, sour, spicy and salty. This relates more to an intrinsic quality rather than actual flavor, although in most cases the two will coincide. For example, sour food includes vinegar, olive and lemon, while spicy food includes green onion, ginger and pepper. Each taste has a different function and works on a specific organ. Therefore one must take care when combining tastes, being sure not to consume too much from one category, creating an imbalance.

TCM treatment is highly individualized, taking into account the specific qualities, as defined by TCM, of both the patient and the medicine. Chinese medicines are composed of plant medicine (roots, stems, leaves and fruits), animal medicine (inner organs, skin, bones, etc.) and mineral medicine. As we will see, tea therapy often uses tea in combination with plant medicine, also called medicinal herbs, taking advantage of the individual properties of each food to treat different diseases.

The prescriptions in this book often contain herbs or foods that may seem exotic, such as astragalus root, wolfberry or ephedra, but are common remedies in TCM. With the growing interest in natural remedies, shops selling these items are now readily found in metropolitan areas in the West as well as being easily found online in most cases.

Now you are ready to begin your exploration of tea therapy!

—*The Editor*

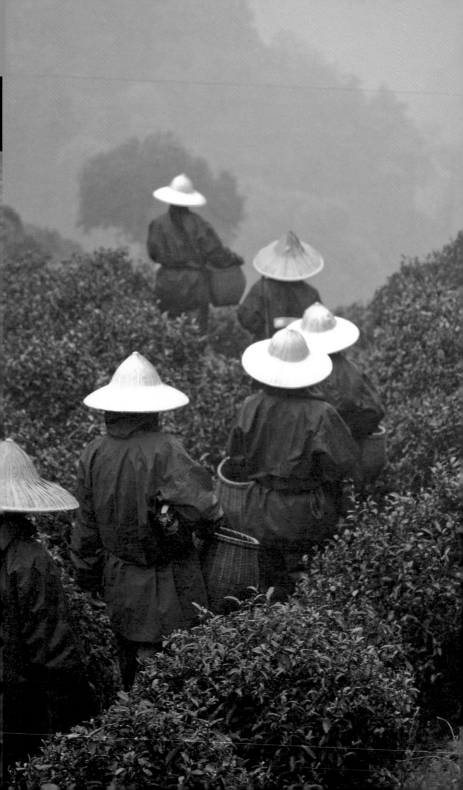

Chapter 1
On Tea

There are three kinds of non-alcoholic vegetal drinks that have been both beloved and popular for thousands of years: tea, coffee and cocoa. The plants from which these three drinks derive are quite different from each other in terms of morphology, zoology, affinity and components. And their sources are on three different continents: Tea trees originate in China, coffee in Ethiopia, and cocoa in the Amazon River and country around Orinoco. But in addition to their popularity, they have in common long histories and many legendary stories. Tea in particular has had a deep and profound influence.

| People are picking fresh tea leaves in the tea garden.

Origin of Tea

The academic name of the tea tree is *Camellia sinensis* (L) Kuntze, which belongs to the Camellia genus of the Theaceae family, according to classifications in botany. Camellia is one of the more ancient members in Theaceae, and tea trees are also comparatively primitive among the species in Camellia.

According to scientific research, tea trees first appeared at the end of Mesozoic Era and the beginning of Cenozoic, or about 70 million years ago. The place of origin is probably the Yunnan-Guizhou Plateau in China, with the heartland being the adjacent zone of the provinces of Yunnan, Guizhou and Guangxi, including the border of the Sichuan Basin.

After having been processed, the buds and leaves of the tea trees can be made into tea. As a kind of evergreen plant, tea trees can grow to a height of more than twenty meters in a wild state. But under the cultivation, they are normally kept around 80 to 120 centimeters in height by pruning, for the convenience of picking the tea leaves.

Tea trees grow best where the temperature is 18 to 25 degrees Celsius, annual precipitation is around 2,500 mm and there is acid soil with certain altitude. The leaves of tea trees alternate in attachment to the stem, and the flowers are white with a pleasant smell. Apart from being planted by sowing seeds, tea trees can also be cultivated with cut-off branches through vegetative

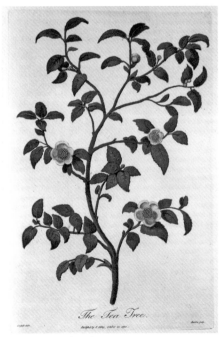

The Tea Tree.

| The illustration of tea plant.

propagation. This latter means has been popularized in recent years since it takes less time for tea trees to form a garden. Usually, it takes five to ten years for a tea tree to become mature, and it can produce tea leaves for about fifty years if it is well managed.

Nowadays, the custom of drinking tea has extended all over the globe and tea trees have become a worldwide cash crop, with the number of countries growing tea trees numbering fifty to sixty. However, China is the source, directly or indirectly, for all tea leaves and tea seeds, as well as for the methods of drinking tea, the art of tea-tasting, cultivation techniques, tea-making technology and tea sets. Therefore, China is the cradle of tea culture. In China, tea culture was first transmitted orally, expanding gradually and then being recorded in books.

Lu Yu and *The Classic of Tea*

Lu Yu (733–804) in the Tang dynasty had a lifelong devotion to tea, and is famous due to his work *The Classic of Tea*, the first monograph on tea in the world. Its publication was of epoch-making significance in the world history of tea. Always respected, Lu Yu became revered as the "Saint of Tea" and even the "God of Tea" by later generations. He once went to 32 prefectures and counties to make investigations into tea, and his footprints can be found in tea zones all over China at that time.

Published in the year 780, *The Classic of Tea* is divided into three volumes and ten chapters, devoting over 7,000 words to the subject. After introducing the origin, properties, name and effects of tea, it then discusses the various tools needed when producing and applying tea; tea-leaf picking and tea making; and the different wares and utensils related to tea drinking. It then covers how to brew and drink tea. Further chapters involve people and literature related to tea issues in the Xia, Shang, Zhou and early Tang dynasties and the kinds of tea in different prefectures. The final two chapters treat tea-making tools and firewood and provide accompanying pictures.

Lu Yu argues for the practice of "shading tea trees with trees on the hillsides facing the sun." This practice has been validated by modern tea science, which has found that planting shading trees in the tea gardens in the south or hillsides facing the sun is beneficial for improving the micro-

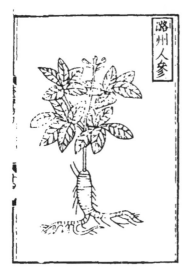 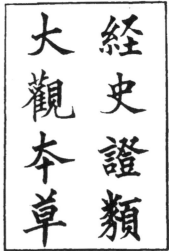

| *Shennong's Materia Medica*

According to ancient Chinese texts, tea leaves had the ability to relieve the symptoms of poisoning. This was first discovered by Shennong in the pre-historic period. *Shennong's Materia Medica* was compiled during the Eastern Han period (25–220). It is the earliest surviving Chinese pharmacological text.

climate in the garden and improving the tea quality.

Lu Yu also proposed the claim that it was "Shen Nong who found that tea is drinkable," referring to the legendary ruler and hero about whom we will learn more later. In *The Classic of Tea*, he quoted one sentence in *Shen Nong's Classic of Food* which had failed to be passed down from past generations: "People who drink tea for a long time can have much vigor and good spirit." This relates to the prevalent notion that "medicine and food have the same source," which has been crucial in traditional Chinese medicine since ancient times.

"Tea-Related Longevity"

It is nature's way for people to be born, grow up and become strong, and then age and die. However since ancient times people have wished for prolonged health and longevity.

In China, people are considered to have a "natural span of life," i.e., there is a standard time limit on a person's life. This is clearly defined in

Yellow Emperor's Inner Canon, the oldest medical text in China: "One passes away according to one's natural span of life and dies at the age of 100 years old." And so it can be seen that a person's maximum age was considered to be around 100 years, which is what we find in surveying long-lived population in modern times or when considering cell division times.

In Japan, if a person lives to 108 years, he or she can be said to have reached "tea-related longevity," a title of honor. This special saying comes from the Japanese character for tea, which was first transmitted from China. If we look at the Chinese character for tea (茶), in the upper part we see two of the character 十 (ten), which represents "twenty"; in the middle is the shape of 人 which when taken apart can be seen as 八 (eight). The lower section is like 木, and can been seen as having 十 (again ten) and 八 (eight), which together become 八十 (eighty). So with the top (20), the middle (8) and the bottom (80), we get 108.

This interesting analysis of the character for tea shows how tea is linked with longevity in people's minds. As supported by its great popularity across a wide range of cultures, tea is truly held as necessary for health and long life. Going all the way back through ancient Chinese literature, we can find people who claim that tea can preserve health and lengthen life, and also people who assert that tea can help get rid of chronic diseases. The health-preserving, anti-aging, and disease-preventing functions of tea have been widely promoted throughout the ages and in different areas of the world.

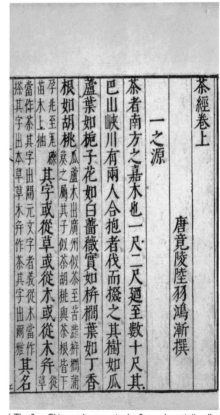

| The first Chinese character in the first column is "tea."

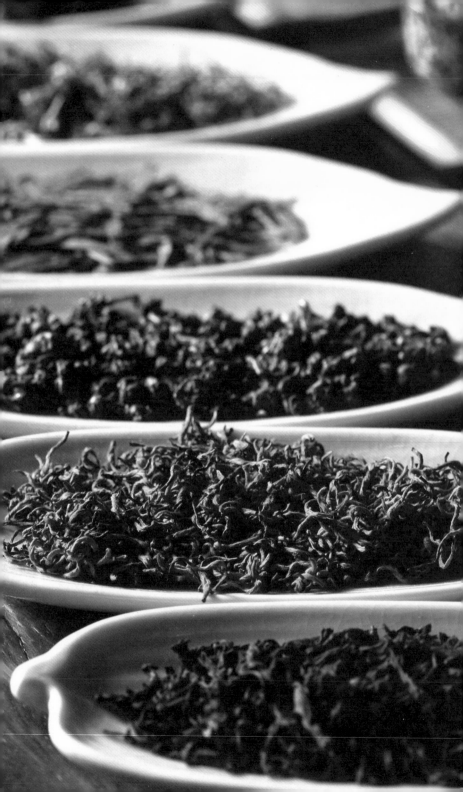

Chapter 2
Tea Therapy

Even though the medical functions of tea have been discussed in more than one hundred works going back to ancient China, the phrase "tea therapy" was never mentioned. At the beginning of the 1980s, I became increasingly interested in the health properties of tea leaves through reading relevant literature and clinical research, and after getting further inspiration from the tea ceremony in Japan, proposed the system of "tea therapy." Tea has numerous effective components and pharmacological functions, and is capable of clinically preventing and treating diseases.

| In China, tea is divided into six categories, namely green tea, black tea, yellow tea, dark tea, white tea and oolong tea.

What Is Tea Therapy?

As the country where tea leaves were first found and used, China has the richest resources of tea trees and its splendid tea culture is famous all over the world. The tea culture that originated in China has developed many other forms under specific historical and cultural conditions found in different countries, and has now spread worldwide.

Tea culture can have very specific formats, for example, the "Jingshan Tea Party," which is a model combining monastic codes and tea etiquette. Popular in Jingshan Temple of Yuhang in China's Zhejiang Province, it includes numerous ceremonial procedures: putting up a tea notice, beating tea drums, respectfully inviting people into the hall, offering incense to Buddha, heating water and whisking tea, taking out small cups and giving out tea, reciting Buddhist verses and drinking tea, finishing the tea, and exiting the hall. The guests and hosts, or the masters and apprentices, talk with each other, or ask and

| *A Literary Party* (detail) by Zhao Ji.
The painting shows the splendor of a Song literary party. The bottom of the painting depicts the preparation of tea with a stove, tea bowls and other utensils, demonstrating the indispensability of tea at this kind of literary function at the time.

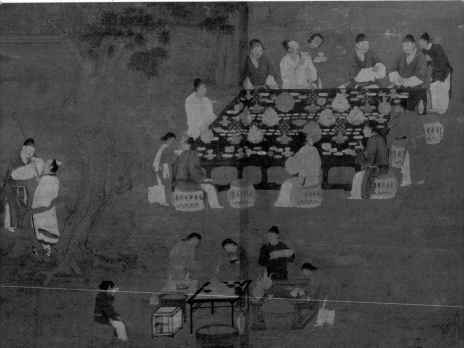

answer questions, with their keen words showing great wisdom. This is a classic style of Chinese Zen-tea culture. After being brought to Japan, the tea ceremony gradually developed further.

Like tea culture, TCM also originated in China. Tea therapy can be seen as a very special branch in the system of TCM treatment. In essence, it can be considered a separate branch in TCM diet therapy, combining TCM and tea culture.

As a kind of traditional Chinese medicine, tea is recorded in works of Chinese materia medica over many centuries. The research on the preventative and curative functions of tea in China started in ancient times. Whenever researching the history of tea in China, one is sure to encounter the character of Shen Nong. According to legend, Shen Nong tasted hundreds of herbs, a story that has been recorded in ancient classics. For example, in the works of the Ming and Qing dynasties, it was written that "Shen Nong experimented with hundreds of herbs and one day he was poisoned with 72 toxins that were cured by tea."

Chen Cangqi, a great medical expert in the Tang dynasty and the author of a book *Gleaning Herbs* whose content is broad and profound, also wrote about the benefits of tea. In *Gleaning Herbs*, he came to an incisive conclusion about the disease prevention and treatment functions of tea: "Tea is the medicine of ten thousand ailments."

I have found that tea therapy is worthy of increased attention and popularity, and generally speaking, has the following six merits:
- reliability (in its curative and preventative effect);
- extensive scope;
- lack of toxicity (which means it can be taken over a long time);
- good taste;
- low price;
- convenience (it needs almost no other special equipment).

In the *Chinese Classic of Tea*, edited principally by Chen Zongmao, the author mentions 23 traditional medical effects of tea, including helping with insomnia, digestion and rheumatic pains, as well as calming nerves, dispelling the effects of alcohol, strengthening teeth and improving eyesight. Contemporary scientific research has discovered additional benefits of tea, in the areas of weight loss, reducing blood fat and blood pressure, preventing and treating arteriosclerosis (including anti-thrombosis), strengthening the heart (including prevention and treatment of coronary heart diseases) and enriching the blood (including increasing white blood cells). It can work against aging, blood sugar, bacteria, inflammation, toxicity and radiation. While the claim that "tea is the medicine of ten thousand ailments" made by Chen Cangqi might be a bit exaggerated, tea clearly has extensive therapeutic effects.

Why does tea have so many rare and beneficial medical effects?

Modern research has analyzed the various components of tea, especially the "effective components," which are also called "active ingredients." Studies have shown that there are twelve major categories of components in tea, with detailed catalogues showing hundreds. Among them, the most important ones are organic chemical components like tea polyphenol, caffeine, amino acids, vitamins, lipopolysaccharides, tea-pigments, aromatic substances and enzymes, as well as inorganic components including phosphorus, potassium, calcium, zinc, selenium and fluorine. Each has its own special curative effect and activity.

Among these, tea polyphenol is the most complicated and the most important. It consists mainly of four components: tea catechins, flavonoids, anthocyanin and phenolic acid. It causes a definite decrease in blood fat while also having an anti-arteriosclerosis effect and improving blood capillary function. In this way, it is useful for prevention and treatment of cardiovascular and cerebrovascular diseases, which are common issues for middle-aged and elderly people. Other important benefits include anti-bacterial, anti-inflammation, detoxification, anti-mutation and anti-radiation effects.

According to TCM theory, each food has its own specific properties and is assigned a "flavor" (which usually but not always relates to its actual taste). In TCM, tea is characterized as sweet, bitter, slightly cold and nontoxic. In TCM, most sweet things help to tonify and most bitter things help to drain or draw out. So tea is a good medicine due to its tonifying and attacking effect.

The attacking effects of tea include clearing heat, removing summer-heat, detoxifying, promoting digestion, removing oil and fat, inducing diuresis, relaxing the bowels, eliminating phlegm, and relieving rheumatic pains among others. The tonifying effects include slaking thirst and helping produce saliva, promoting energy and strength, and prolonging life. Due to its "slightly cold" nature, it has the effects of clearing heat, detoxifying, discharging fire, cooling blood, relieving summer heat and curing boils. Tea therapy takes advantage of these properties, and tea is further beneficial because it is non-toxic, safe and can be taken over a long period of time.

Classification of Tea Therapy

After reviewing literature from ancient times and incorporating modern research, tea therapy can be classified in a broad sense and a narrow sense. Specifically there are three categories of therapy.

Single tea, which means that only one type of tea is used in the remedy, has many effects that other traditional Chinese medicines and Western medicines don't have.

Tea and medicine taken together, based on the compatibility of medicines in TCM, is called "complex prescription of tea therapy." TCM holds that when medicines with similar effects are taken together, those effects can be strengthened, and when medicines with different effects are taken together, the effects can be enhanced or additional benefits created.

Tea substitutes, in which there are actually no tea leaves, may also be used. In this category, traditional Chinese medicines are used in the way of making tea, either by brewing or steeping.

1. Single tea

Of the above-mentioned three types, single tea (single prescription of tea therapy) is the most basic, most important and most appealing. Without this type, there is no possibility of forming any sort of effective tea therapy.

There are many kinds of tea, which is the result of meticulous cultivation by tea growers in different places according to varied climates and soil conditions over the centuries. In the Ming dynasty in China, there were five major types of tea: green tea, black tea, yellow tea, dark tea and white tea. In the Qing dynasty, oolong appeared, giving six basic types of tea. There are additional types, i.e., reprocessed tea, including scented tea (jasmine tea and rose tea, etc.), compressed tea (black brick and cake tea, etc.), and modern and contemporary extracted tea

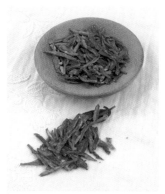

| Longjing tea from Hangzhou.

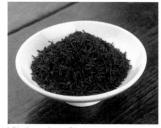

| Black tea from Qimen.

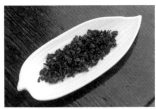

| Oolong tea from Wuyi Mountain.

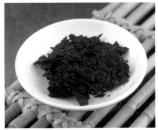

| Pu'er tea from Yunnan.

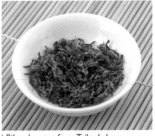

| Biluochun tea from Taihu Lake.

(concentrated tea, and instant tea, etc.), with a total now in the hundreds.

In general, the most important ones are unleavened green tea, leavened black tea and semi-leavened oolong. As for specific varieties, the most famous ones in China include longjing tea (green tea) from Hangzhou, black tea from Qimen, oolong tea from Wuyi Mountain, Pu'er tea from Yunnan, and Biluochun tea from Taihu Lake.

Different kinds of tea have varying curative effects. Among them, oolong tea has quite good curative effects, helping in losing weight, body-building, reducing blood fat, lowering blood pressure, and preventing and treating arteriosclerosis as well as the resultant coronary heart disease and chronic cerebral circulatory insufficiency. The varieties of this type of tea include oolong from northern Fujian Province, such as Wuyi Rock tea; oolong from southern Fujian Province, such as Tieguanyin tea; oolong from Guangdong Province, such as Fenghuang Shuixian tea; and oolong from Taiwan, such as Dongding oolong.

From the perspective of TCM, the nature of green tea is slightly cold while that of black tea is slightly warm. Therefore the type of tea that should be taken can vary according to one's habits or the cold or hot nature of the disease. For example, black tea should be taken for the diseases classified under TCM as "cold" (deficiency-cold or endogenous cold) and green tea for the "hot" diseases. Due to the nature of the disease it is better to take black tea for stomach illnesses like gastric ulcer and chronic gastritis, while green tea is best for enteritis and dysentery, even though both are diseases of the digestive tract.

Green tea is recommended with respect to diet therapy, digestion promotion and oil reduction. Tea leaves also have a therapeutic effect, and after having been soaked they can be dried in the sun and used as stuffing in herbal pillows.

2. Tea and medicine

Also known as the "complex prescription of tea therapy," taking tea and medicine together is also an important kind of tea therapy, second only to single tea. This type of prescription can commonly be seen in medical works in the Tang, Song, Yuan and Ming dynasties. In many monumental works on traditional Chinese medicine, there are special chapters on "herbal tea."

The purpose of matching tea with various traditional Chinese medicines is to strengthen its therapeutic effect in order to treat complex conditions. And there are many purposes for medicine-matching. To enhance curative effects, we can use tea with traditional Chinese medicines that have the same or similar effects. For example, to lose weight or reduce blood fat, you can take tea with water plantain rhizome, lotus leaves and Chinese hawthorn berries, to strengthen these effective properties.

To treat complicated health problems, tea can also be taken with medicine that has a different curative effect. For example, in the traditional Szechwan lovage mixture, tea is used with rhizome of Szechwan lovage (in Chinese *chuan xiong*, also known as Sichuan lovage), which serves to activate blood and promote the circulation of *qi*. This property of the mixture is different from that of tea, but when used together, it can enhance the curative scope and effects of tea (see page 96).

It is a folk practice to often use tea together with food or condiments. The common examples are:

• sugar tea, which can tonify middle *jiao* and *qi* as well as harmonize the stomach and warm the spleen;

• honey tea, which can also tonify the kidney and loosen the bowels, in addition to having the effects of sugar tea;

• salt tea, which can reduce phlegm and reduce heat as well as improve eyesight and promote

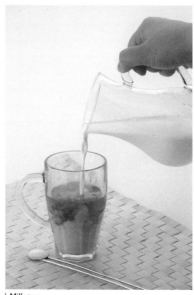

| Milk tea.

purgation;

• ginger tea, which can induce sweat and dispel toxins as well as warm the lungs and relieve cough;

• vinegar tea, which can stop pain and dysentery;

• milk tea, which can nourish the five internal organs (as defined by TCM, namely heart, liver, spleen, lung and kidney) as well as tonify *qi* and produce blood;

• butter tea from the Tibetan minority, which can warm one's body and dispel cold;

• oil tea from the Miao and the Dong minorities, which can strengthen body resistance and eliminate toxins as well as protect against the cold.

3. Tea substitute

In this form of therapy, there is no actual tea used. However the form of drinking tea is adopted, so it is called "tea without tea."

In fact, this therapeutic method dates back to ancient times. For example, according to the description in *On Mengliang*, a classic from the Song dynasty, dried dark plums and fruit of villous amomum soaked in water were sold in tea houses to substitute for tea. So while there is no tea in tea substitutes, it cannot be neglected due to its close relationship with tea drinking since antiquity.

Tea substitutes are steeped or brewed according to the quality of medicine, but it is better to soak those with a "light" nature in hot water while brewing those with a "hard" nature. Most tea substitutes are ones

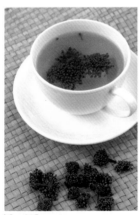

with a light nature; they are mostly soaked in hot water, or even simmered in water, although only for a little while. Generally, the dose is heavy with no distinction between first-time or second-time extraction, and it is consumed frequently without a specific schedule. Condiments can be added to achieve better taste.

Clinically, TCM commonly uses tea substitutes including: chrysanthemum, wild chrysanthemum, flower of pale butterflybush, honeysuckle, herb of christing loosestrife, boat-fruited sterculia seed, folium sennae leaf, mint, herb of fortune eupatorium, herb of

| Sanchi flower tea.

wrinkled gianthyssop, rhizome of lalang grass,

reed rhizome, root of pilose asiabell, root of heterophylly falsestarwort, American ginseng, ginseng, wolfberry, mung bean, tangerine peel, dandelion root or leaf, herb of Manchurian wildginger, rose bud, balloon flower, dendrobium stem, fruit of Asiatic cornelian cherry, safflower, motherwort herb, rhubarb, coptis root, herb of stringy stonecrop, horny goat weed, root of manyprickle acanthopanax, leafy twig of Chinese arborvitae, eucommia bark or leaf, dogbane herb, bamboo leaf, pearl barley, lotus leaf, lotus plumule, leaf of indigowoad, root of Chinese clematis, root of danshen, plantain herb, jujube, and ginger.

Other kinds of tea substitutes, which lie outside traditional Chinese medicine, are those used by people in different regions or cultures. For example, corn silk, pine needle, tender shoots of mulberry trees and sweet-scented osmanthus flowers are used in different areas as tea substitutes. Hawk tea in Sichuan Province uses lauraceae, the tender leaves of which can be dried and taken as tea to relieve summer heat and quench thirst. Sanchi flower tea is a special local product in Yunnan Province, and is used against high blood pressure, acute laryngopharyngitis, hyperlipidemia and coronary heart disease. People in Hangjiahu Plain (located in the northern part of Zhejiang Province) even make tea with salted green beans, to harmonize middle *jiao* and invigorate the stomach.

Historical Development

As for the history of tea application and the question of whether tea was first used as medicine or as a drink, opinions in the academic community differ at present. I believe that tea has been used for about five to six thousand years, and was taken as a drink earlier than it was used as a medicine. In TCM, there is a theory of "medicine and food with the same source" which has many grounds of argument, all claiming that food came earlier than medicine. However it is difficult to completely separate the function of tea as a drink and as a medicine.

The historical development of tea therapy can be divided into the following four periods:

1. Initial period (from the Pre-Qin period to the Han and Jin dynasties)

According to the existing literature, the discovery and application of tea were first recorded around the early Zhou dynasty, which is more than 3,000 years ago. Of course, the practice arose much earlier than the written records. But since tea depended on the emergence of bronze ware or ceramic ware, it cannot be earlier than the early Neolithic Period. So we may say its history is about 5,000 years.

Archaeological studies haven't given a definitive answer. There are many excavated cultural sites of the Shang dynasty (1600–1046 BC), as well as literature handed down from ancient times, but almost none of them are related to tea. People in the Shang dynasty were quite fond of wine, as proven by ancient books and records, inscriptions on bones or tortoise shells and numerous unearthed drinking vessels (which exist in greater quantities even than food containers). Tea is known to dispel the effects of alcohol so we might expect to find references to tea in such a wine-loving culture. However, even though there are many names of plants in Shang dynasty inscriptions on bones or tortoise shells, there are no words about tea. And among the numerous unearthed relics from the Shang, there are no tea wares as such.

Given this lack of archaeological evidence from three to four thousand years ago, this seems to be contradictory to the above-mentioned history of five to six thousand years. But this is actually not the case. This is because, as written by Lu Yu in *The Classic of Tea*, "Tea trees are precious ones in southern China." From studies in paleogeography and paleontology, we can know that tea trees originated from the Yunnan-Guizhou Plateau and the border of the Sichuan Basin. In the Shang dynasty, the population had not spread to that area, so even though there is no proof in records and artifacts that people drank tea, it cannot be claimed that there was no tea usage anywhere at the time in China.

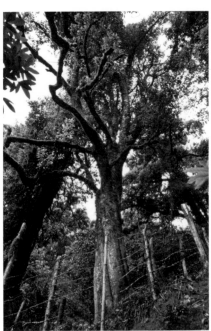

| An ancient tea tree in Yunnan.

What about people in the Zhou dynasty, which followed the Shang dynasty? Geographically speaking, the population in the Zhou dynasty was in Shaanxi Province, which is closer to the birth place of tea than Henan Province, the center for the Shang dynasty. So the dissemination of tea would have been easier; people in the Zhou dynasty likely got tea leaves from Sichuan Province.

As discussed earlier in relation to Lu Yu's *The Classic of Tea* and the figure of Shen Nong, the relationship between tea and Shen Nong has had quite a deep and profound influence. Shen Nong is representative of the agricultural period in primitive society, and there are many things related to Shen Nong in traditional Chinese culture, e.g. tea, medicine, agriculture, diet and ceramics, which in turn are in fact also closely related to each other. As a result, I believe we can say that the discovery and application of tea are related to the "period of Shen Nong" and it was earlier taken as a drink than as a medicine. This is seen in the history of traditional Chinese medicine, and makes sense since medicinal properties can be found after something is eaten, hence the theory of "medicine and food with the same source."

Numerous early medical masters expounded the benefits of tea. Zhang Zhongjing of the Eastern Han dynasty used tea to treat diarrhea and the blood poisoning, pyaemia, writing about it in his *Treatise on Febrile and Miscellaneous Diseases*. Hua Tuo, a highly skilled doctor in the Eastern Han dynasty, used tea to fight fatigue as well as refresh himself. Wu Pu, a well-known doctor in the Wei, a state in the Zhou dynasty, used tea to cure anorexia, stomachache and other ailments, and as a health-care product that could "make one feel at ease and energetic as well and relax one's body and help anti-aging." And it is written in *Guangya* by Zhang Yi in the Wei that "cake tea … helps dispel the effects of alcohol and make one alert."

2. Formation of tea therapy (Tang and Song dynasties)

The Tang dynasty brought theories and practices of tea therapy to the peak, with works such as *The Classic of Tea* by Lu Yu, the first classic in tea science; *Tang Materia Medica* (collectively complied by Su Jing and others), the first record of tea among books on materia medica; and *Gleaning Herbs* by Chen Cangqi, who proposed that "tea is the medicine of ten thousand ailments."

Tea therapy is also recorded in other medical works. For example, the *Supplement to Essential Prescriptions Worth a Thousand Gold* by Sun Simiao, a famous doctor in the Tang dynasty lists "tea, bitter tea" along with content similar to that in *Tang Materia Medica*. In addition, Volume 31 in *Medical Secrets of an Official* compiled by Wang Tao and others specifically talks about a "new prescription of tea substitute," recording the making and drinking methods of tea therapy in detail. *General Records of Holy Universal Relief*, compiled by Zhao Ji in the Song dynasty, records that brewing tea dust and drinking the extraction can cure cholera and anger. Of special note is that, in officially issued monumental great works such as *Peaceful Holy Benevolent Prescriptions*, *Prescriptions of Peaceful Benevolent Dispensary* and *Prescriptions for Universal Relief*, there are special chapters introducing "herb tea" as tea therapy.

While in the Han, Liang and Wei periods, tea therapy was used only as single prescription, in the Tang and Song dynasties, single and compound prescriptions were both developed, with the latter being more prevalent than the former.

3. Development of tea therapy (Ming and Qing dynasties)

In the Tang and Song dynasties, tea therapy became well known in healthcare, having attracted the attention of medical experts, healers and the general public. In the Ming and Qing dynasties, tea therapy was truly in vogue, and application and methods of tea therapy continued to develop. The scope broadened to cover all medical fields such as internal medicine, surgery, gynecology, pediatrics, ophthalmology, otolaryngology, dermatology and orthopedics, having preventative and protective functions.

Among the numerous effective prescriptions that stem from this period are many of those still in common use today, such as: baxian tea (see page 137), ginger tea (see page 79), Szechwan lovage mixture (see page 96), Szechwan lovage tea (see page 141), and pearl tea (see page 137).

During this period, there were comparatively many medical works recording tea therapy in detail. These include *Principles of Correct Diet* by Hu Sihui in the Yuan dynasty, *Compendium of Materia Medica* by Li Shizhen, and *Food Reference to Materia Medica* by Fei Boxiong. In the palace of the Qing dynasty, tea substitutes were extremely prevalent. In *Imperial Medicaments—Medical Prescription Written for Empress Dowager Cixi and Emperor Guangxu with Commentary* compiled by Chen Keji and others, there are nearly fifteen tea substitutes, including one for calming the liver and clearing heat and one for promoting the secretion of saliva or body fluid.

4. Mature period (modern and contemporary)

In contemporary times, with the development of science and technology, there have been numerous discoveries regarding the nutritional components of tea and its medical functions. The curative effects of tea therapy have been further proved by clinical cases. This has led to the increasingly mature status of the field of

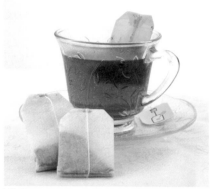

| Tea bags.

tea therapy. Since the 1970s, with the recommendation and use of tea therapy by numerous medical practitioners, the popularity of tea therapy has quietly continued to grow, as various prescriptions of tea therapy have emerged through research and trial.

The application of modern tea therapy has made great improvements from its traditional basis, with the following distinct features:

• Improved dosage form: Tea bags have replaced the traditional way of making tea and have become the prevalent method of tea therapy. Tea is packed in small filterable paper bags to be soaked in boiling water. Easy to make, this kind of tea is also closer to the original in terms of color, smell and taste, with the color being clear without sediments. In addition there have also been scientific developments in making instant tea in the form of a block or crystalline, which is easy to dissolve and absorb as well as convenient and hygienic. Effective constituents in tea, after having been extracted, can be made into oral liquid or tablets.

• Increased range of treatment: Tea can now be used for a wide range of difficult diseases, and for emergent and severe cases. In recent years, medical experts have applied tea therapy to the treatment of such illnesses as diabetes, coronary heart disease, rheumatic heart disease, acute heart failure and impotence.

• International reach: Tea therapy is advancing across the world. Over recent years, TCM has spread its influence in various parts of the world, with more and more people becoming keenly interested in traditional and natural healing methods. Therefore tea therapy, as an important component of traditional Chinese medicine, is also advancing internationally, becoming an accessible family health-care remedy.

Effective Constituents in Tea

The constituents of tea are very complicated. So far, there have been more than 500 compounds that have been separated and identified, among which more than 450 are organic and dozens are inorganic. As proven by modern research, tea has many pharmacological functions, with some realized by a single constituent, some by several constituents, and some through interaction and synergism of different constituents. We will look now at the functions of many constituents of tea.

Constituents Contained in Tea and Corresponding Percentages

Classification		Name	Percentage in weight of fresh leaves (%)	Percentage in weight of dry leaves (%)
Moisture			75–78	
Dry matter (percentage in weight of fresh leaves, 22%–25%)	Inorganic compound	Water-soluble part		2–4
		Water-insoluble part		1.5–3.0
	Organic compound	Protein Amino acid Alkaloid Tea polyphenol Saccharides Organic acid Lipoid Pigment Aromatic substance Vitamin Enzymes		20–30 1–4 3–5 20–35 20–25 Around 3 Around 8 Around 1 0.005–0.03 0.6–1.0

1. Alkaloids

Alkaloids in tea mainly include caffeine (theine), theophylline and theobromine. These three compounds belong to methyl purine and their pharmacologic actions are quite similar.

Comparison of Pharmacologic Actions of Three Alkaloids in Tea

Name	Content in tea (%)	Central excitation	Heart excitation	Smooth muscle relaxation	Diuresis
Caffeine	2–5	+ + +	+	+	+
Theophylline	0.06	+ +	+ + +	+ + +	+ + +
Theobromine	0.002	+	+ +	+ +	+ +

As shown above, it is caffeine that has the main medical effect among the three alkaloids. In every 150 ml tea extraction, there is about 40 mg of caffeine. Caffeine is soluble in water, and usually dissolves in water with a temperature of 80°C. Since it also exists together with tea polyphenol, it differs from caffeine in a free state in terms of physiological function.

In comprehensive evaluations of the safety of caffeine, the conclusion is that with a normal dose, caffeine won't lead to deformity, cancer or mutation. The pharmacological actions of caffeine include: exciting the nervous system, relieving tiredness and improving work efficiency; resisting the toxic action of alcohol, nicotine and morphine, etc.; stimulating the cardiac and vascular systems; increasing renal blood flow, improving filtration rate, and effecting diuresis; relaxing smooth muscle and relieving tracheal and bile duct spasm; controlling the hypothalamus and adjusting body temperature; directly exciting the respiratory center; and promoting digestion.

2. Polyphenols

Polyphenols are a kind of phenol compound with antioxidant properties. Catechins comprise about 70% of the total. So far more than thirty kinds have been found, with their content varying according to the tea variety and preparation.

In green tea, the common content of polyphenols is 15%–35% of the total dry weight, and some even exceed 40%. In black tea, the content is lower (about 10%–20%) since most tea polyphenols will oxidize due to fermentation. In addition to catechins, polyphenols are otherwise composed of flavonoid compounds, anthocyanin and phenolic acid. Of the catechins, the most important are epicatechin (EC), epigallocatechin (EGC), epicatechin gallate (ECG) and epigallocatechin gallate (EGCG), as they are the main active components regarding the curative effects of tea. Catechin has the effects of Vitamin P, and works against radiation damage and migraine.

Flavonoid, also called anthoxanthin, is one of the major components influencing the color of green tea, with the content comprising 1%–2% of the total dry components of tea. Anthocyanin is bitter, so if there is too much anthocyanin, the quality of tea will not be too desirable. It will lead to difficult fermentation of black tea and affect the color of the extraction. A high content of anthocyanin is worse for green tea and will cause bitter and astringent taste as well as dark green waste leaves. The content of phenolic acid in tea is comparatively low, and includes gallic acid, theogallin, chlorogenic acid and caffeic acid. Flavonoid and glycoside have the effect of Vitamin P, promote the absorption of Vitamin C, prevent and treat scurvy, and help with diuresis.

The pharmacological actions of tea polyphenols include: decrease of blood fat and blood sugar; arteriosclerosis control; improvement of blood capillary function; anti-oxidation, control of free radicals and anti-aging; anti-radiation; sterilization and anti-inflammatory effect; alleviation of drug resistance of pathogenic bacteria to antibiotics; and anti-cancer and anti-mutation effects. In recent years, as an antioxidant, tea polyphenol has been widely applied to the food industry and the refined chemical industry.

3. Vitamins

In tea, there are rich vitamins, which are indispensible to health and metabolism. Usually, there are water-soluble vitamins (primarily Vitamin B and Vitamin C) and fat-soluble vitamins (mainly Vitamin A and Vitamin E).

In one kilogram of dry tea leaves, there is usually 100–150 mg Vitamin B. Of the Vitamin B family, the content of Vitamin B_5 (nicotinic acid) is the highest, taking up about half of the total content. A lack of Vitamin B_5 in the body will lead to marked decrease of coenzyme in the liver and muscles, causing illness. Therefore, since tea has comparatively high levels of Vitamin B_5, it is helpful in preventing and curing skin diseases like pellagra.

The content of Vitamin B_1 (thiamine) in tea is also higher than that in vegetables. Vitamin B_1 maintains the normal function of the nerves, heart and digestive system, and promotes the function of glycometabolism. It is important in preventing and curing beriberi, polyneuritis, heart dysfunction and stomach dysfunction.

In every 100 g of dry tea leaves, the content of Vitamin B_2 (riboflavin) is about 10–20 mg. Ailments caused by the lack of Vitamin B_2 can usually be seen in eyes, skin and junctions of mucous membranes, so drinking tea is helpful for the normal function of the retina as well as preventing and curing keratitis, conjunctivitis, seborrheic dermatitis (or inflammation of the scalp), dermatitis and angular cheilitis.

Vitamin B_3 (pantothenic acid) is a kind of complicated organic acid that takes part in many kinds of biosynthesis and metabolic degradation, and helps prevent fatty liver and atherosclerosis (ASVD) as well as preventing and curing dermatitis, trichomadesis and adrenal lesion caused by lack of Vitamin B_3.

The content of Vitamin B_{11} (folic acid) is very high with 0.5–0.7 mg in every kilogram of dry tea leaves. It takes effect in biosynthesis of nucleotide and fat metabolism in the human body.

Another vitamin that exists in high quantities in tea is Vitamin C. In high-quality green tea, the content of Vitamin C can reach as high as 0.5%. Vitamin C is good for the body in many aspects. It can prevent and cure scurvy, improve resistance to organisms, promote healing of wounds, enhance fat oxidation and discharge cholesterol, hence helping prevent and treat arteriosclerosis caused by the increase of blood fat. It takes part in redox reactions in the body, promotes detoxification, and helps to discharge poisonous heavy metal ions. It also has important anti-cancer effects. With a normal diet, three or four cups of good tea taken daily can basically meet the requirements for Vitamin C.

In addition tea contains many fat-soluble vitamins, such as vitamins A, E, and K, which are also important for normal physiological function. The content of carotene in tea is higher than even that of a carrot. It helps in regulating the body, for example by maintaining normal functions of the epithelial cells, preventing keratinization, and taking part in the synthesis of rhodopsin in retina. Vitamin E mainly exists in lipid components. It is a well-known antioxidant, preventing lipid peroxidation, so it has the effect of anti-aging. Vitamin K can promote the liver to combine prothrombin, so it is helpful for the coagulation and hemostasis mechanisms of the body. Five cups of tea can meet the requirements in this aspect.

Even though vitamins exist in relatively large quantities in tea, each tea has different components and ratios. Generally speaking, vitamin content is higher in green tea than in black tea, in high-quality tea over tea of inferior quality, and in spring tea versus summer and autumn tea.

Since fat-soluble vitamins cannot dissolve easily in water, they cannot be easily absorbed or utilized even though the tea is brewed in boiling water. Therefore, other means of "taking tea" are advocated today to make up for this defect, i.e. making tea leaves into ultra-fine powder to add into various kinds of food such as tofu, noodles, pastry, candies and ice-creams. Through these foods containing tea, people can obtain the fat-soluble vitamins, thus better bringing the nutritive value of tea into full play.

4. Mineral substances

There are many kinds of minerals in tea. Among them, the phosphorus and potassium content is the highest, and next comes calcium, magnesium, iron, manganese and aluminum. The micro-constituents include copper, zinc, sodium, sulphur, fluorine and selenium. Most of these minerals are good for human health.

The fluorine content is much higher in tea than in other plants. It has the obvious effect of preventing tooth decay as well as preventing and curing osteoporosis of the elderly.

Selenium is an indispensable constituent of glutathione oxidase (GSH-PX) of the human body. It can stimulate the generation of immunoglobulin and antibodies, strengthen resistance against diseases, help cure coronary heart disease, and control the generation and development of cancer cells. It has been found that Ziyang green tea in Shaanxi Province has a high selenium content. In addition, abundant selenium is contained in tea produced in the area of Enshi in Hubei Province.

Zinc can directly affect the synthesis of nucleic acids and proteins by forming RNA and DNA polymerase as well as the secretion of hypophysis. Hence, lack of zinc may lead to slow growth in children and youngsters and hypogonadism. Zinc can also promote mental functions in both the young and the elderly. The content of zinc in tea is usually 35–50 μg/g.

Iron and copper are both related to the hematopoietic function, or blood production. The content of iron in green tea reaches 80–260 μg/g, and that in black tea 110–290 μg/g. It plays a role in the formation of hemoglobin and in the transportation of oxygen and carbon dioxide in the body. It also takes part in the composition of tissue respiratory enzymes (e.g. cytochrome oxidase and catalase, etc.). Copper can work with iron to promote hemoglobin as a biocatalyst and take part in various kinds of oxidase.

5. Amino acid and protein

Amino acid is the basis of the formation of protein. The content of water-soluble protein that can be directly utilized is only 1%–2%, although this directly affects the taste of tea. Research shows that there are 25 kinds of amino acid in tea, among which theanine is the most abundant, taking up more than 50% of the total of amino acid.

It is well-known that amino acid is necessary for the human body. Some kinds of amino acid are closely related to human health. For example, glutamic acid and arginine can reduce blood ammonia and cure hepatic coma. Methionine can adjust fat metabolism along with other functions. Cystine can promote hair growth and prevent premature senility. Arginine, threonine and histidine can enhance human growth and mental development, improve the absorption of calcium and iron, and prevent osteoporosis.

6. Tea pigments

Pigments in tea include fat-soluble and water-soluble pigments, and comprise only 1% of the total weight of the dry leaves. Water-soluble pigments include flavonoid, anthocyanin, theaflavin (the oxidative product of tea polyphenol), thearubigins, and theabrownin. Fat-soluble pigments (including chlorophyll, lutein and carotene) do not dissolve in water, and they are main constituents to form the color of tea. Especially for green tea, the color and luster of the dry tea, as well as the yellow-green color of waste tea leaves after use, are mainly determined by the chlorophyll content. The color and luster of six kinds of teas (green tea, black tea, yellow tea, white tea, dark tea and oolong tea) are closely related to the specific pigments in them.

7. Other ingredients

Saccharides in tea include monosaccharide, disaccharide and polysaccharide, which comprise up to 20%–25% of the total weight of dry tea leaves. Monosaccharide and disaccharide can dissolve easily in water, and while the content is only 0.8%–4% of the total, they are two of the influences on the taste of tea. Polysaccharide in tea include starch, cellulose, hemicellulose and lignin, the content of which takes up more than 20% of the total dry weight.

There are comparatively many kinds of organic acid in tea, taking up around 3% of the total weight of the dry leaves. Most are free acids such as malic acid, citric acid, succinic acid and oxalic acid. Organic acids generated in the tea-making process include palmitic acid, linoleic acid and ethylene acid, and they are one of the main components of the aroma. About 25 kinds of organic acids have been found in the aroma of tea.

Aromatic substances in tea refer to the volatile substances in tea, and of the total chemical components in tea, they comprise only a small share. In finished products of green tea, aromatic components with comparatively high content are alcohol and pyrazine, mostly generated during the process of drying the green tea leaves. In black tea, the main aromatic components are aromatic compounds of alcohol, aldehydes, ketone and esters, which are oxidized during the processing of black tea.

Enzymes in tea are biocatalysts, taking part in a series of chemical changes that take place during the growth of tea trees and the processing of the leaves. There are many kinds of enzymes in tea. Deactivation of enzymes is a necessary part of the processing course of green tea. The first step is for the fresh-picked leaves to be heated to control fermentation, keep the inherent green color in tea leaves, and decrease the moisture in the leaves to make them softer for further processing. As for fermentation in the processing of black tea, enzymes are activated to reactions that form oxidative products like theaflavin and thearubigins influencing the quality and features of red leaves and red extraction of black tea.

Even though these constituents are not present in large amounts, they have unique curative effects. For example, lipopolysaccharide in tea can resist radiation and increase the number of white blood cells, and compounds of several polysaccharides and diphenylamine in lipid components in tea can reduce blood sugar.

Curative Effects of Tea

The curative effects of tea are quite extensive. In terms of TCM, there are 23 types of traditional effects according to the ancient literature: reducing sleep-time, soothing nerves, improving eyesight, refreshing the mind, slaking thirst and helping to produce saliva, clearing heat, relieving summer heat, detoxifying, helping to digest, dispelling the effect of alcohol, removing grease, lowering *qi*, serving as a diuretic to alleviate water retention, moving the bowels, treating dysentery, removing phlegm, dispelling wind and relieving exterior syndrome, strengthening teeth, treating cardiodynia or heart pain, curing sores and fistula, allaying hunger, benefiting physical strength and prolonging life.

According to modern studies, there are another eighteen curative effects of tea, so there are altogether more than forty, which is indeed rare both in Western and traditional Chinese medicine.

1. Reducing weight

The classification of reducing weight includes decreasing body weight and building up the body. Obesity is usually caused by abnormality in fat metabolism and accumulation of too much fat. Tea helps reduce weight through the comprehensive function of many effective components. Tea polyphenol can dissolve fat, chlorophyll can hinder the digestion and absorption of cholesterol, and Vitamin C can promote the discharge of cholesterol, together leading to an ideal effect of reducing weight.

2. Decreasing blood fat

Decreasing blood fat is the reduction of cholesterol in the blood to prevent and treat hyperlipidemia. Since obesity can often lead to the increase of cholesterol, the effect of tea in reducing weight is also effective for reducing fat. Tea polyphenol can not only dissolve fat, but also control the increase of cholesterol in blood plasma and the liver as well as curb the deposition of cholesterol on artery walls. Therefore, drinking tea daily can not only reduce fat but also prevent the increase of blood fat.

3. Preventing and treating arteriosclerosis

Arteriosclerosis is usually caused by obesity and hyperlipidemia. Many components in tea can work together to reduce weight and fat, and thereby prevent and treat arteriosclerosis to certain extent. In addition, tea polyphenol can restrain hyperplasia of arterial smooth muscle, and help to prevent and treat arteriosclerosis.

4. Preventing and treating coronary heart disease

Coronary heart disease, also called coronary atherosclerosis heart disease, is closely related to the above three kinds of diseases. Statistics have shown that the morbidity of those who don't drink tea is 3.1%, those who occasionally drink tea 2.3%, and those often drink tea (over three years) only 1.4%. The aggravation of coronary heart disease is related to insufficient blood supply to coronary arteries and thrombosis. Animal studies have shown that the tea catechins in tea polyphenol and tea pigment, which are generated by continuous oxidation during the simmering process, improve blood function through anticoagulation, promoting fibrinolysis and anti-thrombosis.

5. Reducing blood pressure

Hypertension means that systolic pressure or diastolic pressure exceeds the normal level. Arteriosclerosis not only leads to coronary heart disease but is also closely related to hypertension. Tea polyphenol and vitamins C and PP in tea are all effective components for preventing and treating hypertension. Of special note is the function of tea polyphenol in improving blood capillary function, and tea catechins compounds and theaflavin in controlling enzyme activity to directly reduce blood pressure.

6. Anti-aging

Lipid peroxidation has been proven to be one of the aging mechanisms in the human body. Antioxidant compounds like Vitamin C and Vitamin E can delay the process. Tea has comparatively large quantities of these vitamins, and tea polyphenol also plays an important role. According to studies conducted by Japanese scholars, the anti-oxygenation of Vitamin E, which is widely regarded as an anti-aging medicine, is only 4%. With its tea polyphenol, green tea's anti-oxidative effect can reach as high as 74%. Moreover, amino acid and microelements in tea also have the function of anti-aging.

7. Decreasing blood sugar

Decreasing blood sugar is important in preventing and treating diabetes. In fact, in Japan, tea was used to create a kind of medicine especially for dealing with diabetes. Clinical studies have shown that tea's effect is similar to that of insulin. Black tea's effect on decreasing blood sugar is inferior to that of green tea, and cold water is better than hot water when used to make tea. So far, three kinds of effective components to decrease blood sugar in tea have been reported: compound polysaccharide, tea catechins compound and diphenylamine. In addition, vitamins C and B_1 in tea can promote metabolism of sugar. Therefore, drinking tea can often be a complementary therapy for diabetes.

8. Controlling bacteria and diminishing inflammation

It has been proved that tea catechins compounds inhibit many kinds of pathogenic bacteria such as typhoid bacillus and paratyphoid bacillus. Flavanol in tea can directly diminish inflammation and promote the activity of adrenal glands, decreasing the permeability of capillaries and decreasing exudation of the blood.

9. Diminishing smoke toxicity

Due to the intake of nicotine, smokers will experience increase of blood pressure, arteriosclerosis and decrease of Vitamin C, which will accelerate aging. It has been shown that smoking one cigarette can reduce 25 mg of Vitamin C in the body, and the concentration of Vitamin C in bodies of smokers is lower than that of non-smokers. Therefore, drinking tea, especially green tea, can help to dissolve smoke toxicity and replenish Vitamin C. Green tea extract can also inhibit many kinds of chemical carcinogens in cigarette smoke.

10. Alleviating toxicity of heavy metal

With the development of modern industry, environmental pollution has inevitably appeared. Excessive levels of various kinds of heavy metals (e.g. copper, lead, mercury, cadmium and chromium) can harm the human body. Tea polyphenol has comparatively strong adsorptive and precipitating effects regarding heavy metal, so tea can alleviate toxicity of heavy metal.

11. Anti-radiation

In studies of rats, feeding black tea, green tea and polyphenols extracted from tea leaves and then exposing them to Radiostrontium-90 (90Sr) of lethal dose, it was found that about 90% can be absorbed by tea and the absorption time is shorter. These results are seen to be applicable to humans.

12. Stimulating the central nervous system

This function of tea is commonly known as refreshing oneself, and it is related to "reducing sleep-time," one of the previously mentioned effects of tea in terms of TCM. Tea can restore consciousness and provide stimulation, helping one's ability to study and strengthening memory.

13. Promoting diuresis

Modern studies show that the main reason why tea promotes diuresis is through the caffeine and theophylline contained in tea. These can increase renal blood flow as well as control mechanisms like water re-absorption of the kidney tubules through expanding capillaries of the kidney.

14. Preventing tooth decay

The function of preventing tooth decay is related to the microelements contained in tea. Old tea leaves have an especially high content of fluorine, which can prevent tooth decay and strengthen bones. In addition, tea polyphenols can kill many kinds of bacteria in the mouth and are effective in treating periodontitis. Therefore, regularly drinking tea or rinsing the mouth with tea can improve oral health.

15. Improving eyesight

Since the eye lenses have a higher demand for Vitamin C than other tissues, if one doesn't have sufficient intake of Vitamin C, the lens will become turbid and can easily be affected by cataracts. Nyctalopia (or night blindness) is mainly related to the lack of Vitamin A. There are high levels of Vitamin C and Provitamin A (i.e., carotene) in tea, so drinking large quantities of green tea can improve eyesight as well as prevent and treat many kinds of eye diseases.

16. Aiding digestion

Caffeine and flavanol compounds in tea can promote alimentary canal peristalsis, helping to digest food and prevent peptic diseases. Therefore, drinking tea after meals, especially after consuming oily foods, is conducive to digestion.

17. Stopping dysentery and preventing constipation

Tea catechins compounds have obvious inhibition effects on pathogenic bacteria. Moreover, since tea polyphenol can enhance intestinal canal peristalsis, drinking tea can also help treat constipation.

18. Dispelling the effects of alcohol

The liver needs Vitamin C as a catalyst to break down alcohol. Drinking tea can replenish Vitamin C and help to detoxify alcohol in the liver. In addition, caffeine in tea, through its diuretic effect, helps to discharge alcohol out of the body, and it stimulates brain function inhibited by alcohol, hence dispelling the effect of alcohol.

19. Other effects

Apart from those mentioned above, tea has many other effects according to data from China and other countries. Tea can prevent the formation of calculus in the gall bladder, kidney, and bladder; prevent and treat various vitamin deficiencies; and prevent hemorrhage and edema in places such as the mucous membranes and gums. Chewing dry tea leaves can alleviate symptoms in pregnant women as well as nausea caused by motion sickness. Moreover dry tea leaves can be used as deodorants to remove the odors such as raw fish and paint. After use, wet tea leaves can be used to boil tea eggs or rub oily furniture and household utensils. Or they can be dried in the sun and stuffed in pillows used to restore consciousness and improve eyesight.

Medicated Diet and Tea Therapy

Diet therapy has an extremely long history and wide range of practice in China. As recorded in the ancient ritual text *Rites of Zhou*, medical science at that time only had three branches, and one of them was "Dietician" (the other two branches were internal medicine and surgery). This serves as the earliest record of medical workers in diet therapy. Dieticians were similar to modern nutritionists who use diet in preventing and treating medical conditions. It incorporates proper food handling and emphasizes what is appropriate to eat or avoid under certain conditions. So it can be seen that in China, people attached great importance to studies and clinical applications of diet therapy from early on.

By modern times, two new branches have derived from diet therapy, one being herbal cuisine and the other, tea therapy. Referring again to the ancient saying "medicine and food have the same source," herbal cuisine makes use of the compatibility of traditional Chinese medicine and food, while tea therapy links TCM with tea or ways of tea-drinking. These two approaches are different but both result in improved health care and disease prevention.

Indeed herbal cuisine and tea therapy can be combined. *The Classic of Tea* by Lu Yu mentioned previously has a story of a woman in the Shu, a state in the Zhou dynasty in southern China, who made and sold tea porridge. Tea leaves can also be added to rice, as in the traditional recipe for "chicken rice with tea flavor," which calls for

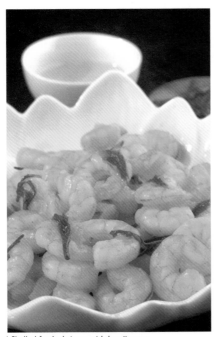

| Shelled fresh shrimps with longjing tea.

the addition of green tea-leaf powder, agar slivers and fine salt.

Tea leaves can be both stir-fried and put into soup. Among stir-fried dishes, shelled fresh shrimp with longjing tea is the most famous, and this dish has spread from Hangzhou to different places in southern and northern China. With its enticing color, aroma and taste, this dish has been favored by both Chinese people and foreigners, and in fact in 1972, when Premier Zhou Enlai entertained President Nixon, during his visit to Hangzhou this dish was served and all the guests praised it.

Other examples of cooking with tea leaves include roasted pork with tea leaves, a famous dish originating with the Confucius family in Shandong Province, as well as duck with camphor tree leaves, a well-known dish in Sichuan. Carp and tea soup in a couple of varieties is also quite common. Other soups include sliced pork soup with longjing tea, and tomato soup with green tea.

Several healthy dishes made with tea are listed here.

1. Thick soup with bean curd, green tea and shrimp

Ingredients: 1 piece of bean curd, 2 g green tea leaves (Qiqiang green tea preferred), 15 g dried shelled shrimp (for preparation: wine, water, salt, MSG, cornstarch, oil).

Preparation: First boil the water, then add bean curd cut into small pieces and the shrimp, which has been soaked in equal amounts of water and wine. Then add wine, salt and monosodium glutamate until the water is again boiling. Skim any floating foam and add the tea leaves. Reduce heat and cook for a while until fragrant. Thicken the dish with mixture of cornstarch and water. Add a bit of chicken oil or salad oil for appearance.

2. Clam and tea soup

Ingredients: 250 g clams, 10 g green tea leaves (longjing tea preferred), ginger.

Preparation: Soak tea leaves in warm water. Put clams and ginger into stockpot with a small amount of boiling water and simmer for a while. Pour the tea in when the shells of the clams begin to open, and wait till the soup is boiling. This soup has a delicious clear broth and tender, fragrant clam meat.

3. Stewed chicken with Tieguanyin tea

Ingredients: one young broiler chicken, 25 g Tieguanyin tea, green onion, ginger, sugar.

Preparation: Soak Tieguanyin tea in hot water. Cut the broiler chicken into big pieces. Put the pieces into an oiled pan and fry them till half-cooked. Add green onion, shredded ginger and Tieguanyin tea. Use high heat until the tea water boils, then reduce heat and simmer, adding a little sugar at the end. Note: Duck and pork ribs can be stewed in the same way.

How to Drink Tea

Though tea therapy has many merits, it cannot be said to be without shortcomings. The curative effects of tea therapy depend on how people apply it, and if it is properly used, many of these shortcomings can be avoided. The following section outlines some of the elements that can influence tea therapy's effectiveness.

1. Constitution

The concept of "constitution" is pivotal to TCM, and therefore to tea therapy. TCM holds that different methods should be used depending on your constitution type. Under TCM, symptoms may present as cold or hot, and medicine also can be classified by qualities of warmth and coolness. These concepts do not refer to the actual surface temperature but the inherent nature.

The nature of tea leaves is complex. Normally they are classified as slightly cold, but black tea made after fermentation becomes slightly warm. There are numerous other examples like this in TCM, for example the nature of ginseng after being steamed (which is called red ginseng) is warmer than that of common ginseng (sun-dried ginseng).

Therefore, using the theory of TCM, tea should be taken discriminately, i.e., according to one's constitution or the nature (cold or hot) of the disease. In terms of constitution, people with cold or cool constitutions are better off taking black tea (classified as warm or hot), while those with warm or hot constitutions benefit from green tea (classified as cool or cold). Regarding the nature of the disease, for digestion-promotion and grease-removal, green tea is more appropriate, while for diabetes, hyperlipidemia or fatty liver, oolong tea is the best choice since these diseases are considered damp-phlegm according to TCM.

2. Seasonal changes

In traditional Chinese culture, there is a theory called "correspondence between man and universe." Humans are influenced by their external surroundings, so the different seasons affect methods of health care. Under this belief, since drinking tea is one of the ways to maintain health, it should also vary according to different seasons.

As stated earlier, generally the nature of black tea is believed to be hot and green tea cold. Green tea contains more tea polyphenol than black tea, and the taste is more bitter. According to TCM, it is often said that if a medicine tastes bitter, then its nature is cold. This underlies the concept that green tea has a cold nature and black tea a hot nature.

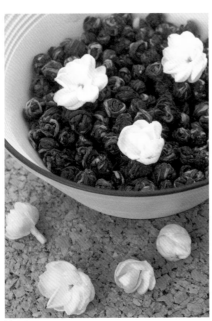

| Jasmine tea.

Accordingly, you can arrange your tea-drinking plan according to seasons based on the nature of the tea. Drink scented tea in spring and autumn because it is warm and fragrant. Green tea is best for summer, and you can also add some chrysanthemum, honeysuckle, lemon juice or mint to green tea to strengthen the effect of relieving summer heat. Drink black tea with sugar or milk in winter to harmonize the stomach and warm your body. This basic plan will vary from person to person according to temperament and interest, and of course, some people prefer to drink the same kind of tea no matter the season.

3. Type of diseases

In tea therapy as in most treatments, it is important to use the appropriate prescription for the disease. For example, it is better to drink black tea for stomach illnesses (e.g. chronic gastritis) and green tea for intestinal problems (enteritis and dysentery) even though they are both related to the digestive tract.

Even within the broad categories, care must be taken to treat specific conditions. For example, ulcers are a type of stomach ailment, a category for which black tea is normally recommended. However, it has been proven that drinking tea can increase hourly maximal acid output (MAO), which can accelerate the emergence and development of ulcers. Therefore, people with ulcers or those who are suspected of having ulcers, should avoid by all means drinking strong tea. They should only drink light black tea with a proper amount of milk and sugar.

In another example, tea can prevent and treat coronary heart disease, but when the caffeine level reaches certain amount, it will lead to acceleration of the heartbeat. So patients with coronary heart disease, featured by evident premature heartbeat, tachycardia and atrial fibrillation, must avoid drinking too much tea or strong tea.

Drinking tea is good for the health, but taking in too much caffeine in tea can cause such reactions as the increase of blood cholesterol, insomnia, headache and depression. And some may have tachycardia and even cardiac failure, which was called "tea intoxication" in ancient times. Patients with chronic heart disease, end-stage cirrhosis and some weakened elderly people should drink tea in moderation, and it is better for them to take light tea. Patients with diabetes can only take some old tea with little caffeine. Moreover, when people participate in evening events, drinking too much tea will cause insomnia, affecting the ability to work the next day. For patients with insomnia, tea is normally forbidden at night.

4. Dietary habits

The quantity and type of tea taken is influenced by what people eat. Since tea has the traditional function of removing fat, people who eat a lot of fatty food should drink tea. Salted vegetables like pickles as well as cured meat products like bacon, ham and sausage often contain high levels of nitrate, and vegetables stored for a long time will generate secondary amine, as will mold contamination in pickled food. When there are both nitrate and secondary amine in food, they can cause chemical reaction and generate nitrosamine, a dangerous blastomogen, which can easily cause cell mutation and result in cancer. Tea catechins can block synthesis of nitrosamine, so after eating pickled vegetables and cured meat products, people should drink a lot of high-quality green tea with a comparatively high content of tea catechins so as to control carcinogens and enhance immune function.

5. Gender and life-stage

Women who are pregnant or breast-feeding should control tea drinking. Studies on mice have shown that a dose (20 mg/kg) of longjing tea can lead to early development delay and behavioral change. Even though this dose is equivalent to a human drinking about 21 cups of tea per day, it should still be heeded. Therefore, pregnant women and breast-feeding women had better not drink strong tea, and in addition tea has the function of astringency, which will lead to decreased breast milk.

Light tea taken by children can replenish some minerals such as vitamins, potassium and zinc. An appropriate amount of tea can improve gastrointestinal function and help digestion in children, since drinking tea can clear and decrease heat and prevent dry stool. The fluorine content in tea is comparatively high, so drinking tea or rinsing the mouth with tea can prevent tooth decay. Taking a proper amount of tea can also help with focus and concentration in children, as it can help regulate their nervous system. Tea also has many other effects like promoting diuresis, protecting against infection and reducing inflammation. Given these benefits, it is acceptable for children to drink tea, but it is best that they do not take strong tea.

6. Appropriate time

It is not appropriate to drink too much tea before or after meals. Too much tea before meals will dilute digestive juice and reduce appetite. Too much tea after meals will increase the burden on stomach since the alkali in tea will neutralize gastric acid, and its water will dilute gastric juice, hence prolonging the time needed for digestion. In the long run, the stomach will be harmed and health will be influenced. In tea there is tannic acid that can bond with the protein and iron in food, thus affecting their digestive absorption in the body. This can lead to growth retardation and anemia. Generally speaking, it is not appropriate to drink tea within one hour after meals.

7. Appropriate tea

While there are many varieties of tea leaves, there is also variety in tea depending on the age of the leaves. Traditionally it has been said that "fresh tea is precious" while "old wine is valuable." But studies have shown that people should not drink too much fresh tea too hastily. There are two reasons: Firstly, the aroma of fresh tea hasn't reached its peak, and there are some aromatic substances in tea that can only be tasted after having been stored for a period of time. Secondly, there are unoxidized and unconverted aldehydes and alcohols in fresh tea, which may have some side effects.

8. Taboos

People often ask whether they can drink tea made during the previous night, and there is a common saying, "tea of the previous night cannot be taken." The problem is not about whether the tea is made on the previous night or not, but rather how long ago the tea has been made. The problem is related to whether the container or storage environment is clean or not, and whether there is sourness, staleness or bacterial pollution or not. Of course, under normal conditions, it is natural to avoid drinking tea made a long time ago. In addition to hygienic factors, this may be related to polonium, a radioactive substance. Polonium is retained in tea leaves after having been soaked for eight hours; the longer the soaking time, the more that will be leached out.

Generally speaking, it is not appropriate to take medicine with tea. TCM states that tea cannot be drunk while taking such medicines as ginseng, root of pilose asiabell, root of Chinese clematis and others. The same applies to Western medicine: Tea cannot be taken with such drugs as iron supplements and ephedrine. The consequences may vary from reducing the drug's effect to causing adverse side effects like vomiting and hiccupping.

To sum up, the shortcomings of tea therapy can be reduced to a minimum as long as people drink tea properly. They must understand their bodies and their ailments thoroughly, and pay attention to the variety (green tea, black tea, oolong tea, etc.), quality (light tea versus strong tea) and quantity of tea.

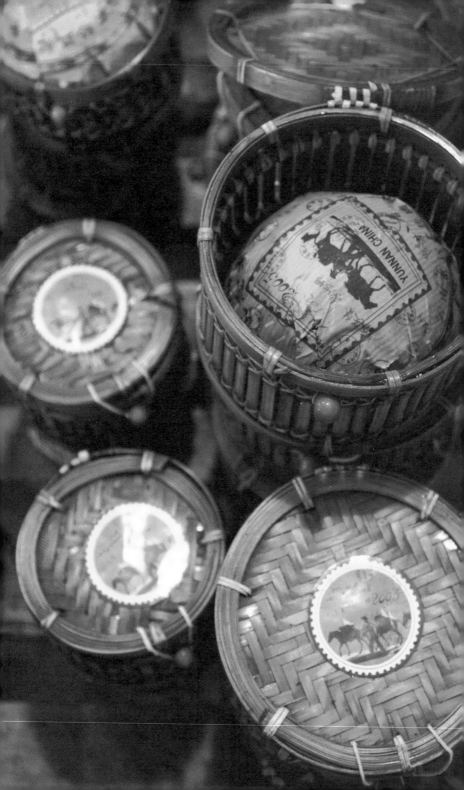

Chapter 3
Preventing and Treating Cardiovascular Diseases

It is widely acknowledged that cardiovascular diseases seriously affect human health. There have been tremendous changes in lifestyle and dietary structure in modern times, and lack of activity, over-eating and poor nutrition have led to various kinds of cardiovascular diseases with complicated causes.

| Unique to Yunnan Province in China, Pu'er tea has a desirable effect of easing high blood pressure and other cardiovascular diseases.

Obesity and Weight Reduction

Obesity refers to too much fat accumulated in the body, and generally speaking, if one's weight exceeds the average by 10%, one is said to be extremely fat, while exceeding by 20% is defined as obese. Obesity is mainly related to the following factors: consuming too many calories; genetic factors; not burning enough calories; and diseases particularly those affecting the endocrine system and fat metabolism.

In recent years and across the world, there seems to be one craze after another aimed at reducing weight. There are many ways to lose weight, e.g. diet control, exercises and drugs. Due to the comprehensive effect of many active components in tea, it can lead to reduced weight and lowered lipids. Reducing weight by drinking tea is the most natural and effective method.

For example, gymnema tea (which has the nickname "sugar-killer") can effectively restrain the absorption of sugar. After chewing its leaves, one will not sense sweetness when taking sugar. This leads to a natural decrease in the intake of food, hence the absorption of sugar and carbohydrates will be lower and the transformed fat mass will decrease correspondingly. Gymnema tea is not only effective for preventing obesity and losing weight, but also has an auxiliary therapeutic function for diabetes.

The reason why tea has the desirable and popular effect of reducing weight is related to many effective components contained in its extraction, with the most important ones being tea polyphenol, vitamins and amino acid. These components have a remarkable effect on fat metabolism, being capable of decomposing fat, removing cholesterol deposited in blood vessels, and discharging them out of the body through urine.

Vitamin C has a special role in promoting the discharge of cholesterol, and tea catechin can prevent the accumulation of cholesterol and help cleanse the blood and liver. Sterol and spinasterol can adjust fat metabolism and reduce cholesterol in blood. Chlorophyll in green tea can also reduce cholesterol by inhibiting it from being digested and absorbed, which is different from and complementary to the functions of tea polyphenol and Vitamin C.

Various kinds of tea have the effect of reducing weight, with especially famous ones being oolong tea, Pu'er tea and longjing tea. Nowadays, there are a large number of weight-reducing teas produced as a means of traditional Chinese medicine. The below three teas are very effective in controlling weight.

Dark tea: When speaking of obesity, people will immediately think of abdominal fat, and dark tea has a definite effect in controlling the accumulation of abdominal fat. Dark tea is produced through the fermentation of *Aspergillus niger*. Just as its name implies, its color is dark. In the fermentation process, a certain component will be generated to prevent fat accumulation. To lose weight by drinking dark tea, it is best to drink strong tea that has just been made. Drink 1.5 liters daily, with one cup before and one cup after meals, and make this practice part of your daily routine.

Lotus leaf tea: In ancient times, drinks made with the flowers, leaves and fruit of the lotus were noted to not only make people feel refreshed, but also help improve complexion and reduce weight. Making full use of lotus leaf tea to reduce weight requires some little tricks. First of all, the tea should be strong because the effect of the second infusion is not very good. Secondly, the tea should be drunk many times per day, with a complete dose finished each time. Thirdly, the tea should be taken on an empty stomach, the benefit of which lies in reduced consumption of food. Lotus leaf tea will help relieve constipation, which is helpful for reducing weight. After drinking this tea for a while, the appetite will naturally change and one won't feel like eating oily food any more.

Oolong tea: This is a kind of semi-fermented tea, which contains almost no Vitamin C but is rich in minerals such as iron and calcium, and also contains components that promote enzyme digestion and fat decomposition, helping to burn the fat in the human body. In semi-fermented tea, there is diuretic caffeine and small amounts of such substances as theophylline, alkaloid and oxalic acid, which promote fat metabolism, helping to reduce weight. Drinking a cup of oolong tea before and after a meal can enhance the decomposition of fat, causing it to be directly discharged from body without being absorbed, thereby preventing obesity caused by intake of too much fat.

1. Pu'er tea

Ingredient: 6 g Pu'er tea.

Procedure: Simmer it for 5 minutes with fresh water, or put it in a cup and infuse with boiling water for 10 minutes.

Usage: It is to be taken warm whenever you like.

Efficacy: It invigorates the spleen to promote digestion as well as remove oil and fat. In addition to treating obesity, it is mainly taken for nausea and vomiting, cough with copious whitish viscid sputum, and to clear toxins in the body.

2. Compound oolong tea

Ingredients: 3 g oolong tea, 18 g pod of Japanese pagoda tree, 30 g Chinese cornbind, 18 g peel of Chinese waxgourd, 15 g Chinese hawthorn berries.

Procedure: Simmer the last four ingredients together in water for 20 minutes. Then use the extracted liquid to soak the oolong tea.

Usage: It is to be taken whenever you like.

Efficacy: It is mainly taken for obesity and hyperlipidemia, as it has the function of removing oil and reducing weight. It also nourishes the liver and kidney, nourishes and darkens hair, and helps in keeping fit and lengthening one's life.

3. Bottle gourd tea

Ingredients: 3 g tea, 15 g dried peel of old bottle gourd.

Procedure: Grind together into rough powder and infuse with boiling water.

Usage: It is to be taken whenever you like.

Efficacy: It has the effect of reducing weight.

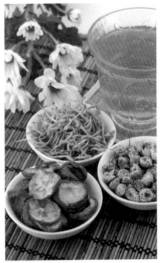

| Hawthorn and flower tea.

4. Hawthorn and flower tea

Ingredients: 10 g Chinese hawthorn berries, 10 g honeysuckle, 10 g chrysanthemum.

Procedure: Smash the Chinese hawthorn berries and then simmer everything together in water.

Usage: You may frequently drink this tea substitute.

Efficacy: It removes stasis and fat, as well as cools and depressurizes. It is mainly taken for obesity, hypertension and hyperlipidemia.

5. Mulberry twig tea

Ingredient: 20 g tender mulberry twigs.

Procedure: Cut the tender mulberry twigs into thin slices, and infuse with boiling water for 10 minutes.

Usage: Drink often.

Efficacy: According to TCM, it has the effect of expelling wind-damp and moving water and smoothing *qi*. It is mainly taken for obesity and arthralgia.

6. Lotus leaf and hawthorn tea

Ingredients: 60 g lotus leaves, 10 g Chinese hawthorn berries, 10 g pearl barley, 5 g balloon flowers.

Procedure: Grind into fine powder, then infuse with boiling water.

Usage: Drink often.

Efficacy: It has the effect of

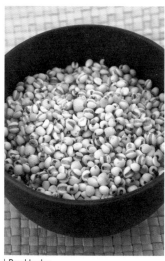

| Pearl barley.

recuperating *qi* and moving water, as well as decreasing blood fat and breaking down turbid and oily substances. It is mainly taken for simple obesity and hyperlipidemia.

Hyperlipidemia

Hyperlipidemia can be divided into three types according to the different blood fat components that show abnormal changes: hypercholesteremia, hypertriglyceridemia and combined hyperlipidemia.

Hyperlipidemia is one of the important factors leading to arteriosclerosis, especially hypercholesteremia. If the amount of cholesterol in blood can be controlled well, the possibility of coronary arteriosclerosis can be effectively decreased.

The lipid-lowering function of tea has received recognition both in ancient and modern times. "Dissolving thick oil," "removing grease" and "rid human fat" are among those properties of tea recorded in ancient literature obviously related to lipid-reduction.

Why can tea-drinking reduce blood fat and cholesterol? This is mainly because there is a great deal of tea polyphenol (especially tea catechin) and Vitamin C in tea. Polyphenol compounds can dissolve fat and are very important for fat metabolism. Tea can not only markedly restrain the increase of blood plasma and cholesterol in liver, but also promote discharge of lipid compounds from the body. Vitamin C can also promote the discharge of cholesterol. Chlorophyll in green tea can not only destroy the cholesterol in food, but also that which is circulating in the intestines and liver, reducing overall cholesterol levels in the body.

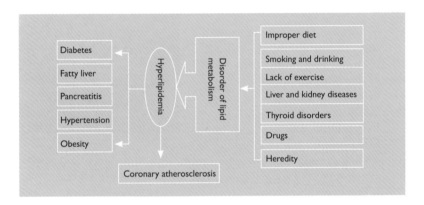

1. Three-treasure tea

Ingredients: Equal amounts of Pu'er tea, chrysanthemum and momordica fruit.

Procedure: Grind these three ingredients into rough powder, and divide into small packages weighing 20 g. Infuse with boiling water.

Usage: Drink it as a tea substitute once a day.

Efficacy: It has the effect of depressurizing, removing oil and reducing weight, as well as preventing and treating hypertension, hyperlipidemia, and headache and dizziness caused by hyperactivity of liver-*yang*.

2. Persimmon leaf and hawthorn tea

Ingredients: 10 g persimmon leaves, 12 g Chinese hawthorn berries, 3 g tea leaves.

Procedure: Soak them in boiling water for 15 minutes.

Usage: Frequently drink this kind of tea substitute.

Efficacy: It has the effect of promoting blood circulation to remove blood stasis, depressurizing and reducing fat, as well as preventing and treating coronary heart disease, hyperlipidemia and hypertension.

3. Cassia seed cholesterol-lowering tea
Ingredient: 30 g cassia seeds.
Procedure: Simmer in water.
Usage: Take twice per day, once in the morning and once in the afternoon.
Efficacy: It can reduce serum cholesterol, and is mainly taken for hyperlipidemia, hypertension and arteriosclerosis.

4. Chinese cornbind medley tea
Ingredients: 20–30 g Chinese cornbind, 20 g Chinese taxillus (the twigs and leaves), 10 g rhizome of Solomon's seal, 6 g honey-fried licorice root.
Procedure: Simmer together in water.
Usage: Frequently drink this kind of tea substitute.

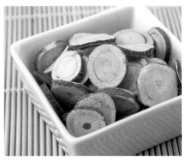

| Licorice root.

Efficacy: It is mainly taken for coronary heart disease of the middle-aged and elderly, as well as to decrease blood fat.

5. Hawthorn and Chinese cornbind tea
Ingredients: 60 g Chinese hawthorn berries, 30 g Chinese cornbind.
Procedure: Simmer in water.
Usage: Frequently drink this kind of tea substitute.
Efficacy: It is mainly taken for hyperlipidemia.

6. Hawthorn and malt tea
Ingredients: 60 g Chinese hawthorn berries, 30 g crude malt.
Procedure: Simmer in water.
Usage: Frequently drink this kind of tea substitute.
Efficacy: It is mainly taken for hyperlipidemia.

7. Five-leaf gynostemma tea
Ingredient: 30–50 g herb of five-leaf gynostemma.
Procedure: Simmer in 1,000 g of water for 15 minutes. Drink the tea only.
Usage: Drink this tea substitute several times. Or add 15 g of

five-leaf gynostemma herb to make tea, drink it, and add hot water again. Repeat until the tea becomes tasteless, and then you can discard the herb.

Efficacy: It has the effects of moving *qi* and nourishing blood, eliminating bruises and wounds, removing obstructions and enhancing immunity, as well as preventing diabetes, neurasthenia and hyperlipidemia.

8. Lingzhi mushroom tea
Ingredients: 10 g lingzhi mushroom, 20 g honey.
Procedure: Simmer lingzhi mushroom in water, and add honey.
Usage: Drink warm, as a tea substitute.
Efficacy: It has the effects of tonifying deficiency, helping one to keep fit and soothing the nerves. It is mainly taken for coronary heart disease, hypertension and hyperlipidemia.

Atherosclerosis

Atherosclerosis is quite harmful, especially for the elderly, but adults in their prime and even youngsters can also suffer from this disease. More men suffer from this disease than women, and the former usually have a more severe state of illness. City dwellers, people in high-stress positions, those that are overweight or smokers, and those having hypertension, diabetes and hyperlipidemia are more likely to be affected by this disease.

Tea polyphenol can improve the permeability of the walls of blood capillaries, effectively enhance the elasticity and resistance of the myocardium and vascular wall, and lessen the degree of atherosclerosis. Vitamins C, B_1, B_2 and PP in tea can reduce cholesterol as well as prevent and treat atherosclerosis. Other kinds of vitamins are related to oxidation and increased metabolism of harmful substances.

Caffeine and theophylline in tea can directly stimulate the heart, expand coronary arteries, strengthen myocardial functions, help to reduce weight and fat, and prevent and treat atherosclerosis. Pigments in tea can influence antithrombin and fibrinolysis activity, reduce platelet adhesiveness and alleviate hypercoagulability caused by atherosclerosis.

Oolong tea, green tea and Pu'er tea are more helpful for preventing and treating arteriosclerosis than other kinds of tea. In addition to drinking tea, to prevent and treat this disease, people should eat properly to prevent weight gain; avoid eating too much animal fat; eat more fresh vegetables, fruits, beans and other bean products; and choose soya-bean oil and vegetable oil when using oil. They should also take part in appropriate sports activities.

1. Banana and honey tea

Ingredients: 50 g banana, 10 g green tea leaves, a little honey.

Procedure: First soak tea in a cup of boiling water, then peel the banana and mash it, adding it with honey to the tea.

Usage: Frequently drink this kind of tea substitute.

Efficacy: It depressurizes as well as having a moistening and laxative effect. It is mainly taken for arteriosclerosis, coronary heart disease and hypertension.

2. Fat-removing fitness tea

Ingredients: 15 g scorched Chinese hawthorn berries, 8 g lotus leaves, 5 g rhubarb, 10 g Chinese angelica root, 10 g rhizome of oriental water plantain, 15 g astragalus root, 2 slices of ginger, 3 g licorice root.

Procedure: Simmer together in water for extraction.

Usage: Frequently drink this kind of tea substitute.

Efficacy: It has the effects of moving *qi* and removing fat, relaxing the bowels and dispelling accumulated and stagnant material. It helps reduce weight in conjunction with an exercise program. It is mainly taken for hyperlipidemia, arteriosclerosis, hypertension and obesity.

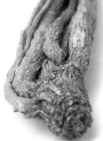

| Chinese angelica root.

Coronary Heart Disease

Coronary heart disease is caused by atherosclerosis of the coronary arteries, the vessels that provide blood flow to the heart.

Excessively high blood cholesterol, hypertension and smoking are the main causes of coronary heart disease and are called primary danger factors. In addition, lack of physical exercise, being overweight, and having diabetes, mental stress and family history of coronary disease can all affect the morbidity of this disease and lead to early age of onset. These factors are listed as secondary danger factors.

Tea has the effects of anti-coagulation and preventing blood clots. The attributes listed in the above section on atherosclerosis are also relevant regarding coronary heart disease: Tea polyphenol can improve the permeability of blood capillary walls, effectively enhance the elasticity and resistance of the myocardium and vascular wall, and lessen the degree of atherosclerosis. Caffeine and theophylline in tea can directly stimulate the heart, expand coronary arteries, and strengthen myocardial functions. Vitamins C and P can also improve the functions of blood capillaries and promote discharge of cholesterol. According to studies, a kind of sour tea polysaccharide can decrease blood pressure, slow down heart rate and enhance the function of the flow of the coronary arteries.

For the above reasons, drinking tea is indeed effective for coronary heart disease. But one should be patient, and especially not overdo tea drinking in the hope of gaining its benefits quickly. It is better to drink light tea than strong tea to prevent heartbeat accelerations, which will aggravate the heart's workload. Generally speaking it is better to drink green tea and oolong tea.

1. Vinegar tea
Ingredients: 8 g tea leaves, rice vinegar.

Procedure: Grind tea leaves into a fine powder and mix with rice vinegar.

Usage: One dose, twice daily.

Efficacy: It has the effects of clearing away heart heat, dispelling depression and relieving pain. It is mainly taken for cardiodynia and it is especially good for those with fire stagnation.

2. West Lake tea
Ingredients: 6 g longjing tea leaves, vinegar.

Procedure: Simmer longjing tea leaves in water and use the extraction. It is better not to simmer it for too long; it is ready when the water begins to boil. Mix with vinegar.

Usage: This makes one dose, which you can separate into several portions to take over the course of a day.

Efficacy: It lowers *qi* and removes stagnant substances, as well as dispersing stasis and relieving pain. It is mainly taken for chronic cardiodynia.

3. Danshen root tea
Ingredients: 9 g root of danshen, 3 g green tea leaves.
Procedure: Grind the root into rough powder, and put it in boiling water with tea leaves for 10 minutes.
Usage: It can be taken whenever you like.
Efficacy: It has the effects of activating blood, removing stasis and relieving restlessness. It can prevent and treat coronary heart disease and angina pectoris.

4. Blood-activating tea
Ingredients: 5 g safflower, 5 g sandalwood, 1 g green tea leaves, 25 g brown sugar.
Procedure: Simmer together in water and use the extraction.
Usage: Separate extraction into two doses, and take one in the morning and the other in the afternoon.

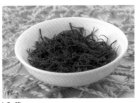

| Safflower.

Efficacy: It has the effects of promoting blood circulation to remove stasis, reducing blood pressure and blood fat as well as expanding vessels. It is mainly taken for coronary heart disease, hypertension and cerebral thrombosis.

5. Ophiopogon tuber tea
Ingredients: Ophiopogon tuber.
Procedure: Simmer it to make extraction.
Usage: Take 10 ml per time (including 25 g crude drug), three times per day.
Efficacy: Frequently drinking this tea can improve myocardial nutrition, enhance hypoxia tolerance of the myocardium, and withstand myocardial ischemia and infarct. It is mainly taken for coronary heart disease, and by middle-aged and elderly people at risk for, or suspected of having, coronary heart disease.

6. Heart-health flower tea
Ingredients: 15 g tea leaves, 6 g flowers of large-flower jasmine,

1.5 g jasmine, 6 g rhizome of Szechwan lovage, 1 g safflower.

Procedure: Bake the rhizome of Szechwan lovage and safflower till they become yellow. Then grind them and mix with other ingredients. Pack them into separate bags of filter paper.

Usage: It is to be taken throughout the year.

Efficacy: It has certain effects for chest distress, palpitation, sleeplessness and uneasiness at night, dizziness and headache.

7. Chrysanthemum and hawthorn tea

Ingredients: 10 g chrysanthemum, 10 g Chinese hawthorn berries, 10 g tea leaves.

Procedure: Infuse with boiling water.

Usage: Frequently drink this kind of tea substitute.

Efficacy: It has the effects of clearing heat, helping digestion and invigorating the stomach, and reducing fat. It is mainly taken for hypertension, coronary heart disease and hyperlipidemia.

8. Sanchi flower tea

Ingredients: 3 g dried Sanchi flowers.

Procedure: Infuse with boiling water, and soak in the warm water for a while.

Usage: Frequently drink this kind of tea substitute.

Efficacy: It is beneficial for people with coronary heart disease, hyperlipidemia and chronic liver disease.

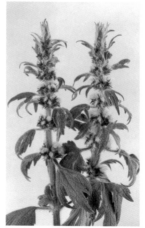

| Motherwort herb.

9. Hawthorn and motherwort herb tea

Ingredients: 30 g Chinese hawthorn berries, 10 g motherwort herb, 5 g tea leaves.

Procedure: Infuse with boiling water.

Usage: Drink it as a tea substitute.

Efficacy: It eliminates phlegm by cooling, activates blood, reduces fat and invigorates the pulse. It is mainly taken for coronary heart disease and hyperlipidemia.

10. Lobed kudzuvine combination tea

Ingredients: 15–18 g crude root of lobed kudzuvine, 18 g root of danshen, 9 g wolfiporia extensa (a fungus also known as Tuckahoe or Indian bread), 6 g licorice root.

Procedure: Take ten of the above portions of ingredients and grind together. To make one dose, take 40 g of the mixture and put it into a thermos bottle. Infuse with half a bottle of boiling water, and cover it for 20 minutes.

Usage: Drink it as a tea substitute.

Efficacy: It has the effects of delivering nutrients to the head and eyes, promoting the secretion of saliva or body fluid, activating blood and reducing phlegm. It is mainly taken for coronary heart disease, oppressive pain in the cardiac area, as well as pain in the shoulder and back.

11. *Yang*-activating tea

Ingredients: 9 g bulb of longstamen onion, 9 g snkaegourd fruit, 4.5 g prepared pinellia rhizome, rice wine.

Procedure: Take ten of the above portions of the first three ingredients and grind together. For a single dose, take 20–40 g of the mixture and put it into thermos bottle. Infuse with half a bottle of boiling water and 10 ml rice wine, and cover it for 10–20 minutes.

Usage: Frequently drink this kind of tea substitute.

Efficacy: It has the effects of relieving chest distress, activating *yang*, removing stasis and relieving pain. It is mainly taken for obstruction of *qi* in the chest and cardiodynia. Those with deficiency of *yin* and deficiency of vital energy should take it with caution.

Hypertension

Hypertensive disease comes in two forms. Primary hypertension is a chronic medical condition in which blood pressure is elevated. Secondary hypertension is caused by other conditions that affect the kidneys, arteries, heart or endocrine systems. As the most common cardiovascular disease, primary hypertension is a serious threat to human life and health. It has been called "a silent killer" by the World Health Organization.

According to studies, drinking tea can reduce the possibility of suffering from hypertension. Regularly drinking more than 120 ml of green tea or oolong tea per day for more than a year leads to a 40% decrease in hypertension when compared with those who don't drink tea. Many effective components in tea leaves can prevent and treat cardiovascular diseases of various kinds (e.g. by reducing fat, improving vessel function, and so on).

Tea leaves can also indirectly reduce pressure through ridding the body of excess fluid and sodium. The effects of diuresis and sodium discharge are two or three times better through drinking tea than by drinking water, because there is caffeine and theophylline in tea.

In tea, there is also rutin, which helps to enhance elasticity of capillaries and prevent increase of blood pressure that may result in hemorrhage. Flavonoids like compounds of flavanol in tea can improve resistance and elasticity of the blood capillary wall to a great extent and enhance the assimilation of Vitamin C.

In relation to hypertension, controlling the activity of angiotensin I converting enzyme can help to reduce blood pressure. It has been proved that tea catechin compounds (especially ECG and EGCG) and theaflavin in tea can inhibit this enzymatic activity. Tea catechin in strong tea can also help to depressurize, while caffeine can directly reduce pressure by relaxing blood vessels. Aminophylline in tea can expand vessels to increase circulation and help to reduce blood pressure. Vitamin PP can expand small vessels to directly reduce pressure.

Various kinds of tea can prevent and treat hypertension, some of the most important of which are described in this section.

1. Cape jasmine fruit tea

Ingredients: 30 g very fresh tea leaves, 30 g fruit of cape jasmine.

Procedure: Simmer together in water.

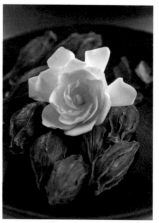

| Fruit and flower of cape jasmine.

Usage: Drink it as a tea substitute.

Efficacy: This tea will purge intense heat, remove heat from the liver, cool blood and reduce pressure. It is mainly taken for hypertension, headache and dizziness.

2. Flower green tea

Ingredients: 3 g chrysanthemum, 3 g flowers of Japanese pagoda tree, 3 g green tea leaves.

Procedure: Put ingredients in a cup and infuse with boiling water.

Usage: Drink often.

Efficacy: It has the effect of calming the liver, dispelling wind, clearing heat, and relieving pressure as well as headache caused by hypertension, fullness in the head, and dizziness.

3. Tall gastrodia tuber tea

Ingredients: 6 g tuber of tall gastrodia, 3 g green tea leaves, honey to taste.

Procedure: Simmer gastrodia tuber with a large amount of water for 20 minutes, and then add green tea leaves. Take the extraction and add honey to it.

Usage: One dose daily, divided into two portions taken at different times, warm.

Efficacy: This tea will calm the liver and suppress *yang*, dispel wind and stop pain, as well as relieve hypertension, headache and dizziness.

4. Eucommia leaf tea

Ingredients: Eucommia leaves and green tea leaves.

Procedure: Grind equal amounts of eucommia leaves and green tea leaves into rough powder, mix them, and put the mixture into separate small packages, each weighing 6 g.

Usage: Drink once to twice per day, one package each time, infused with boiling water.

Efficacy: It has the effect of nourishing the liver and kidney, and strengthening bones and muscles. It is mainly taken for hypertension and heart disease as well as backache and soreness around the waist. Components in eucommia leaf can promote metabolism and heat consumption, and reduce neutral fat, thus reducing body weight. These components can prevent aging and build up the body.

5. Oolong chrysanthemum tea

Ingredients: 3 g oolong tea (or longjing tea) leaves, 10 g chrysanthemum.

Procedure: Infuse with hot water.

Usage: Drink as a tea substitute.

Efficacy: This prescription is applicable to hypertension marked by hyperactivity of liver-*yang*, or *yin* deficiency and *yang* excess. This tea should not be too strong, or insomnia and acceleration of heartbeat may occur.

6. Hawthorn and lotus leaf tea

Ingredients: 15 g Chinese hawthorn berries, 12 g lotus leaves.

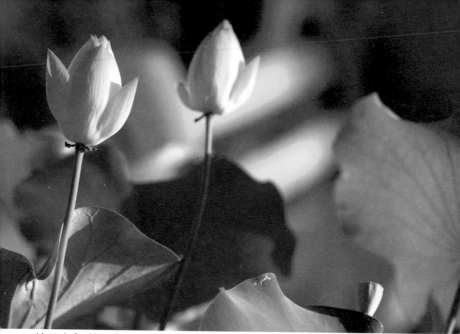

| Lotus leaf and lotus flower.

Procedure: Chop and simmer in water or infuse with boiling water.

Usage: Use the strong extraction as a tea substitute.

Efficacy: It has the effect of reducing fat, generating body fluid, and helping to reduce pressure and weight. It is mainly taken for hypertension, hyperlipidemia and obesity.

7. Lobed kudzuvine tea for hypertension

Ingredients: 30 g root of lobed kudzuvine, 15 g flower buds of Japanese pagoda tree, 15 g motherwort fruit.

Procedure: Simmer or soak together in water.

Usage: Drink it as a tea substitute.

Efficacy: It can treat hypertension.

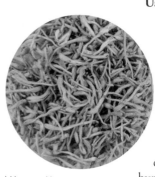

| Honeysuckle.

8. Honeysuckle chrysanthemum tea

Ingredients: 24–30 g chrysanthemum, 24–30 g honeysuckle.

Procedure: Infuse with boiling water.

Usage: Drink as a tea substitute.

Efficacy: It has the effect of antibiosis, antiphlogistic, eyesight improvement and depressurization. It is mainly taken for hypertension and coronary heart disease.

9. Persimmon leaf tea

Ingredient: 30 g fresh and tender persimmon leaves (or 15 g dry persimmon leaves).

Procedure: Infuse with boiling water.

Usage: Drink as a tea substitute.

Efficacy: This tea will help in enhancing resistance against invasive organisms as well as prevent and treat various kinds of diseases, primarily hypertension and coronary heart disease.

10. Chinese taxillus tea

Ingredient: 20 g Chinese taxillus (the twigs and leaves).

Procedure: Simmer in water.

Usage: Drink the extraction, twice a day.

Efficacy: It can treat coronary heart disease and angina pectoris, and is helpful for auxiliary treatment for hypertension.

11. Liver-calming and heat-clearing tea

Ingredients: 1.8 g Chinese gentian, 1.8 g vinegar root of Chinese thorowax, 1.8 g rhizome of Szechwan lovage, 3 g chrysanthemum, 3 g dried rehamnnia root.

Procedure: To make the vinegar root of Chinese thorowax, mix slices of the root with vinegar (50 g root of Chinese thorowax requires 6 g vinegar). Put in a pan and fry on low heat until the vinegar is gone and the root slices are a bit dry. Then dry the slices further in the sun. When the root is ready, mix together with the other ingredients, turn into powder and simmer in water.

Usage: Drink as a tea substitute.

Efficacy: It has the effect of clearing heat, calming the liver, nourishing *yin* and activating the blood. It can treat early-stage hypertension.

12. Evergreen tea

Ingredients: 6 g evergreen tea leaves, 6 g chrysanthemum, 6 g mulberry leaves, 6 g rhizome of lalang grass, 6 g branch of gambir plant.

Procedure: Simmer all ingredients in water.

Usage: Drink extraction as a tea substitute.

Efficacy: Useful for clearing heat, reducing pressure and curing hypertension.

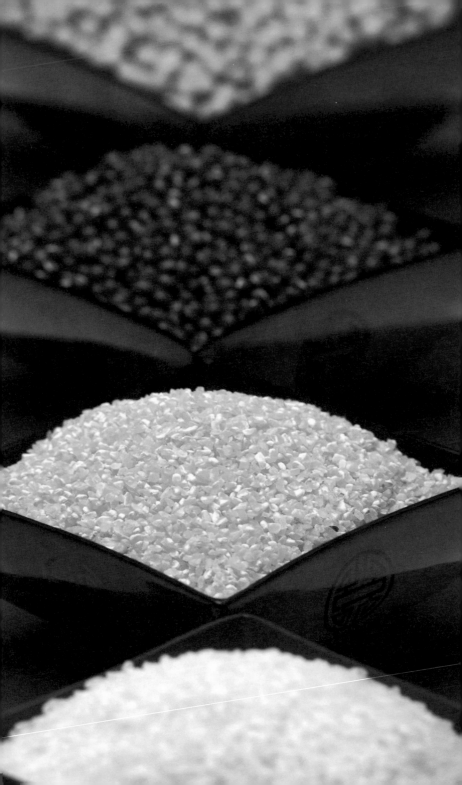

Chapter 4
Adjusting the Nervous System

Diseases of the nervous system stem from many different origins, both genetic and environmental. Often complex to categorize and treat, they all exert tremendous influences on everyday life. The following section lists several common symptoms, which can be alleviated by different means of tea therapy.

| Tea therapy is conducive to adjusting the nervous system. Grains, such as rice, red beans and mung beans, can be used as ingredients in the prescription.

Lassitude

The simple effect of refreshing and energizing oneself may have been the earliest recognized of the many medical benefits of tea.

Since it is a taboo for monks to doze off in the temple, they have long relied on tea to give themselves a lift. They often plant tea trees around the temple and most of them drink tea. It is commonly understood that drinking tea can provide refreshment, increase mental sharpness and eliminate fatigue. It has been so since ancient times.

Following the well-known Chinese saying of "savoring Zen in tea," a cup of tea taken after high-stress work will immediately lift one's spirits and alleviate tiredness. And tea can indeed improve work efficiency greatly. As just one example, in an experiment, after drinking 100 mg of tea, a typist increased his typing speed by 5%–10% with obviously fewer mistakes.

According to modern studies on physiology, even though fatigue stems from a wide range of reasons, it is mainly caused by the central nervous system, especially the activity of higher nerves. In cases of low mood and sleep insufficiency, people will easily feel tired. Tea can refresh oneself as well as stimulate and improve the functions of central nervous system, so people will not feel tired after taking tea. For people who get up too early or work at night, drinking tea can keep their mind clear and get rid of drowsiness.

Apart from factors of the nervous system, theophylline in tea can neutralize acidosis of muscles, improve muscle strength and thus help get rid of tiredness. And in addition to fighting fatigue and stress, tea can also cure many pathological diseases, such as drowsiness and coma caused by disease.

There are two sides to be considered. If tea is properly used as a refreshing stimulant, it is of course beneficial, but under certain conditions, it also has side effects. For example, some people cannot drink tea at night since it makes it difficult to fall asleep. Moreover drinking too much tea can lead to insomnia, palpitation, cardiodynia and blurred vision. Therefore, tea has different effects on different people, so each person must understand "when to say when" in relation to drinking tea.

1. Szechwan lovage and scallion tea

Ingredients: Tea leaves, rhizome of Szechwan lovage, white scallion.

Procedure: Simmer in water.

Usage: Drink it as a tea substitute.

Efficacy: It is taken for phlegm-heat (generated due to abnormal accumulation of human body fluid) and lethargy.

2. Cortex albziae flower and jujube tea

Ingredients: 1 g green tea leaves, 15 g cortex albziae flowers, 25 g jujubes.

Procedure: Simmer in 350 g of water for 3 minutes.

Usage: Split into two portions to drink at different times. Make sure to eat the jujubes.

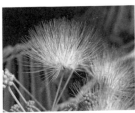
| Cortex albziae flower.

Efficacy: It is taken for melancholia.

3. Five-taste tea

Ingredients: Tea leaves, dried ginger, salt.

Procedure: Mix the ingredients and soak them with boiling water. Add some cooked beans and black (or white) sesame.

Usage: Drink it as a tea substitute.

Efficacy: It can help to remove coldness, generate heat, stimulate one's appetite, eliminate tiredness and treat cold and weakness. After a day of stressful work, if you feel fatigue and low spirits, a cup of this strong tea is recommended to take the tiredness away immediately.

4. Rice tea

Ingredients: 6 g old tea leaves, 50–100 g rice.

Procedure: Simmer tea leaves first, and then use the extraction to make rice porridge (congee).

Usage: Take it warm twice daily, once in the morning and once in the afternoon.

Efficacy: It helps rid the body of drowsiness and fatigue, so it is better not to take it before going to bed.

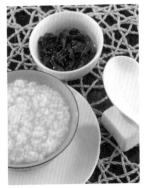
| Rice tea.

5. Schisandra berry tea

Ingredients: 1 g green tea leaves, 4 g schisandra berries, 25 g honey.

Procedure: First fry berries until slightly scorched. Then soak the above ingredients in 400–500 ml boiling water.

Usage: Split into three portions and finish over the course of the day, taking it warm.

Efficacy: It is taken for neurasthenia, tiredness and drowsiness.

Neurasthenia

While the term "neurasthenia" is rarely used these days in Western medicine, in traditional Chinese medicine it remains a valid diagnosis with a set of symptoms and causes. It is a kind of neurosis disorder that is mainly demonstrated by excitability, chronic fatigue and mental lassitude, anxiety, and difficulty in falling asleep. Some patients even have symptoms of headache, dizziness, blurred vision, tinnitus, palpitations, difficulty breathing, erectile dysfunction, premature ejaculation or menstrual disorder. Generally speaking, patients with neurasthenia usually have enduring emotional stress and psychological pressure prior to the onset of the disease.

According to the theory of Pavlov, neurasthenia is mainly caused by the weakening of two processes of inhabitation and excitation within the cerebral cortex. Caffeine contained in tea leaves can enhance the excitation function, and a small amount of it can also improve the process of inhibition. Therefore, it can treat neurasthenia, especially weak-type neurasthenia (marked by insomnia at night and low spirits during the day). Drinking a proper amount of tea during the day and take some calming drugs are quite effective for this.

Some patients with neurasthenia are afraid of drinking tea because of insomnia, believing that tea will serve as a stimulant, thus aggravating the illness. This concern is totally unnecessary because if they drink tea during the day, it will not affect nighttime sleep, but strong tea is still contraindicated.

For a topical application, one can take tea leaves that have been already soaked in water, dry them in the sun, and then add a little jasmine (or chrysanthemum). Mix them evenly and stuff them into a pillow. It can treat neurasthenia, and has such effects as reducing heat, lowering pressure, relieving heat, improving eyesight, and relieving dizziness.

1. Ginger tea

Ingredients: Ginger and tea, ground into very small pieces (fannings).

Procedure: Soak in water.

Usage: Drink it as a tea substitute.

Efficacy: It is taken for discontentment or restlessness, after cholera.

2. Ginseng and semen ziziphus spinosa tea

Ingredients: 5 g ginseng, 15 g wolfiporia extensa, 10 g semen ziziphus spinosa.

Procedure: Simmer in water.

Usage: Frequently drink this tea substitute.

Efficacy: It has the effects of nourishing the heart, tonifying *qi* and soothing the nerves. It is mainly taken for anxiety, fright and palpitations.

3. Sleep aiding tea

Ingredients: 10–20 g common rush.

Procedure: Simmer it for extraction.

Usage: Drink this tea substitute once a day, warm, 1 to 2 hours before sleep.

Efficacy: It can soothe nerves, clear away agitation, relieve restlessness, treat insomnia and irritability, and reduce night-time disturbance in children.

4. Lotus plumule tea

Ingredients: 2 g lotus plumule, 3 g licorice root.

Procedure: Soak in boiling water.

Usage: Frequently drink it as a tea substitute.

Efficacy: It is taken for discontentment or restlessness, and sleeplessness caused by accumulation of internal heat.

5. Common rush and bamboo leaf tea

Ingredients: 5 g common rush, 30 g fresh bamboo leaves.

Procedure: Grind together into powder and simmer in water.

Usage: Drink it as a tea substitute.

Efficacy: It is taken for asthenic fever (a fever with muscle weakness), discontentment or restlessness, and insomnia.

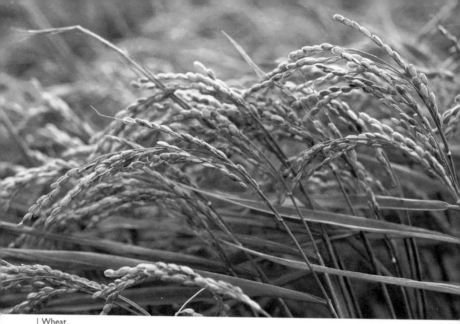

| Wheat.

6. Nardostachys rhizome tea
Ingredients: 18 g nardostachys rhizome, 4.5 g tangerine peel.
Procedure: Soak in 500 ml of boiling water. Leave in water for 3 hours, bringing to boil once every half hour.
Usage: Divide into 12 doses, taking it 6 times per day. Drink it as a tea substitute.
Efficacy: It is taken for neurasthenia, gastrointestinal spasm and stomachache caused by nerves.

7. Licorice root, wheat and jujube tea
Ingredients: 30 g wheat, 10 jujubes, 6 g licorice root.
Procedure: Simmer in water.
Usage: Drink it as a tea substitute.
Efficacy: It is mainly taken for absent-mindedness, lethargy and inability to act on one's own, and sadness, caused by cardiosplenic deficiency.

Headache

The quick tempo of modern life has forced people to devote themselves to stressful work and study. Headache has become an extremely common ailment. Among patients with headache, most are white-collar workers and females. Headache can result from sleep insufficiency, mental fatigue, rage, irregular lifestyle and excessive pressure. In China, dating back to *Prescriptions Worth a Thousand in Gold*, a famous medical book in the Tang dynasty, the benefits of tea are noted, with the saying that it can "cure cracking-like headache."

Tea is ingenious in terms of its curative and preventative effects. Tea can cure headache by soothing nerves and calming people on the one hand, and on the other, through its Vitamin P, can enhance the function of blood vessels on the other. Moreover tea has the effects of anti-freezing and anti-platelet aggregation, so it can be seen as a prophylactic of vascular headache.

1. Rhubarb tea

Ingredients: Rhubarb and tea leaves.

Procedure: Grind rhubarb into fine powder. To make one dose, take 3–5 g of rhubarb and 3 g of tea leaves and soak in boiling water. Drink when warm.

Usage: Take once or twice a day.

Efficacy: It has the effects of clearing heat, curing faintness, purging intense heat, and relieving pain. It is mainly taken for headache caused by reversed flow of qi due to internal heat.

2. Fructus viticis tea

Ingredients: 6 g fructus viticis.

Procedure: Simmer fructus viticis in water.

Usage: Drink as a tea substitute.

Efficacy: It can cure wind syndrome of the head.

3. Dahuriae angelica root and chrysanthemum tea

Ingredients: 9 g root of dahuriae angelica, 9 g chrysanthemum.

Procedure: Grind them into fine powder and put in a vacuum flask. Infuse with boiling water and cover for 15 minutes.

Usage: Drink it as a tea substitute. One dose per day.

Efficacy: It has the effects of dispelling wind, clearing internal heat and relieving pain. It is mainly taken for:

• headache, dizziness, fever with aversion to cold, nasal obstruction, hoarseness, aching limbs and by patients confirmed to have caught a common cold due to wind-cold;

• chronic migraine that comes on intermittently. It is contraindicated for those with deficiency of *yin* and blood heat.

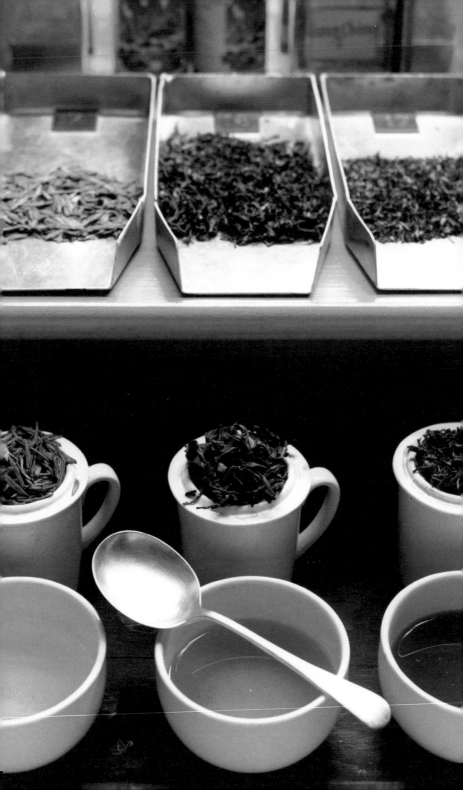

Chapter 5
Protecting the Digestive System

There are many written records about the function of tea in helping digestion. While opinions differ regarding the meaning of an ancient saying in China that "a simple diet can prolong life," it may refer to supporting the digestive system through drinking a lot of tea and taking in less fat and oil to increase health and longevity. Tea has been proven to help digestion and regulate fat metabolism, and in a broad sense, through helping digestion it is beneficial to the entire digestive system.

| Various teas have a curative effect on the digestive system. The liquid resulting from different tea leaves is diverse in appearance.

Dyspepsia

The method of using tea to treat indigestion (or dyspepsia) and abdominal distension dates back to the Qing dynasty. The most beneficial aspects of tea in helping digestion are removing grease as well as the odor of mutton and seafood.

When eating fatty meat, drinking tea is recommended. This makes tea a necessity for people of ethnic minorities from the border area of China, who have fatty meat as a central part of their diet. Tea is taken for oily food and that with a fishy smell as well as for the heat from highland barley.

The effect of tea on the digestive system is complicated and multifaceted. Theophylline can relax the smooth muscle of the stomach and intestines, and reduce pain caused by spasm in the gastrointestinal tract. Catechin can activate enzymes related to digestion and absorption, as well as promote the growth of helpful microorganisms and discharge of hazardous substances through the intestinal tract. Caffeine can stimulate gastric secretion, benefit digestion and enhance appetite. It can also combine with organic acid and other salts, becoming not only more soluble in water but also less aggravating for the mucous membrane. Other components adjust fat metabolism, most prominently vitamins such as inositol, folic acid and pantothenic acid; others include methionine, lecithin and choline.

While tea helps promote digestion, it also has the function of stopping hemorrhage caused by gastric ulcer. This is because polyphenols in tea can attach to the wound of stomach, creating a film to protect it. This function also applies to the treatment of intestinal and gastric fistula.

Different kinds of tea can help digestion in varied ways. It is generally believed that it is better for patients with gastric diseases to take black tea.

1. Jasmine combination tea
Ingredients: 6 g jasmine, 6 g rhizome of grassleaf sweetflag, 10 g oolong tea leaves.

Procedure: Remove any foreign materials from the above, and then dry or warm them for a little while. Soak in boiling water for 5–10 minutes.

Usage: Drink once daily as a tea substitute.

Efficacy: It is taken for chronic gastritis, poor appetite, dyspepsia, abdominal fullness and distension, anxiety and depression, and insomnia and dreaminess.

2. Licorice ginger tea

Ingredients: 1–2 g black tea leaves, 3–5 g dried ginger, 3 g honey-fried licorice root.

Procedure: Wash the ginger, cut it into slices and dry. Put ingredients together in a cup with a cover, add 300 ml of water, and soak them for 5–10 minutes.

Usage: One dose per day, divided into three portions to take after meals.

Efficacy: It has the effects of warming the stomach, dispelling cold and preventing vomiting. It is mainly taken for stomach cold, vomiting, aversion to cold, and thin, watery stool.

3. Digestion-promoting combination tea

Ingredients: 3 g wrinkled gianthyssop, 6 g fortune eupatorium, 5 g mint, 1.5 g fruit of round cardamom (without peel).

Procedure: Grind into powder, and soak in a covered state for 10 minutes.

Usage: One dose per day. Drink it as a tea substitute.

Efficacy: It is taken for promoting digestion, relieving dyspepsia and activating appetite. It is effective for those who have eaten too much fatty food, have indigestion or lack of appetite, feel greasy or tasteless in the mouth, or have bad breath or acidic odor in the mouth after waking up.

| Mint.

4. Hawthorn berry and tangerine peel tea

Ingredients: 20 g Chinese hawthorn berries, 5 g tangerine peel.

Procedure: Fry the Chinese hawthorn berries on low flame. Cut the tangerine peel into pieces. Soak them together in water.

Usage: Drink it as a tea substitute.

Efficacy: It can treat indigestion, loss of appetite, and retention of food.

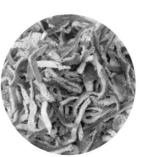

| Tangerine peel.

5. Ginger and pinellia rhizome tea

Ingredients: 10 g ginger, 7 g prepared pinellia rhizome, brown sugar.

Procedure: Wash the ginger and squeeze for its juice. Decoct the prepared pinellia rhizome with water for 5–8 minutes, taking the clear liquid and mixing it with ginger juice. Add a little brown sugar.

Usage: Drink it as a tea substitute. One dose, split into 3–4 portions to take over the course of a day. Take it continuously for 3–5 days.

Efficacy: It reduces phlegm and prevents vomiting. It is mainly taken for gastric asthenia (muscle weakness) and bloating caused by indigestion, frequent vomiting, saliva or phlegm cough.

6. Roasted malt and hawthorn berry tea

Ingredients: 10 g roasted malt, 3 g roasted Chinese hawthorn berry flakes, brown sugar.

Procedure: Put in a cup, add about 250 ml of water, and cover the cup for 20 minutes.

Usage: Drink it as a tea substitute when it is warm, 2–3 doses per day.

Efficacy: It has the effect of promoting digestion to eliminate stagnation. It is mainly taken for dyspepsia caused by excessive eating or improper diet, abdominal fullness and distention, belching with fetid odor, acid regurgitation, vomiting (especially after meals, of undigested food with acidic odor), white coating of the tongue, and unhindered pulse (smooth pulse, as defined by TCM).

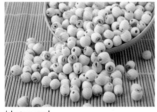
| Lotus seed.

7. Lotus seed tea

Ingredients: 30 g lotus seeds, 30 g brown sugar.

Procedure: Soak lotus seeds in warm water for 5 hours, then stew them with brown sugar till they become tender.

Usage: Add tea and drink it.

Efficacy: It has the effect of tonifying the spleen and stomach. It is especially suitable for those with nephritis and edema to drink it every day.

8. Dried persimmon tea

Ingredients: 6 pieces of dried persimmon, 15 g rock candy (or large sugar crystals), 3 g tea leaves.

Procedure: Stew dried persimmons until they are tender, and add rock candy and tea.

Usage: Drink it as a tea substitute.

Efficacy: It has the effects of regulating the flow of vital energy, easing the removal of obstructions, reducing phlegm, benefiting the intestines and invigorating the stomach. It is best for patients with tuberculosis to drink.

Over-Consumption of Alcohol

Drinking tea benefits the digestive system in many ways, and one of them is dispelling the effects of alcohol. This doesn't mean merely alleviating or dispelling a hangover, but getting rid of the toxicity of alcohol, the meaning of which is deeper.

Since tea polyphenol, theophylline, caffeine, xanthine, flavonoid, organic acid and many kinds of amino acids and vitamins in tea coordinate with one another, tea is a prescription to dispel the effects of alcohol, in particular working together with certain herbal medicines. Its main functions are: stimulating the nervous system, counteracting the inhibiting effect of alcohol to lessen the sense of lightheadedness; expanding blood vessels to benefit circulation and discharge alcohol from the blood; and improving the capability of liver metabolism. It also promotes quick discharge of alcohol through the diuretic effect, expanding the capillaries of the kidney and inhibiting re-absorption by kidney tubules, thus dispelling the effects of alcohol.

However, on occasion, drinking tea after serious drunkenness can cause problems. Taking strong tea immediately after getting drunk will irritate the kidney, which is already under pressure. Moreover, drinking too much tea with excessive water can also burden the heart and kidney, which is harmful to people suffering from high blood pressure and coronary disease.

For the sake of your health, never drink too much liquor, and don't drink too much tea after getting drunk. Of course, a cup of nice tea after drinking liquor is conducive to reducing the effect of liquor and improving digestion of food. In China, it is a habit for families to take tea after a banquet.

In general, it is advisable to apply tea-drinking to reduce the effect when drinking small or moderate amounts of alcohol, but it is not appropriate to do so if drinking heavily. Various teas have desirable functions regarding reducing the effect of liquor.

1. Disintoxicating tea
Ingredients: 60 g tangerine peel, tea leaves.
Procedure: Dry the tangerine peels by a fire, and add a few tea leaves. Decoct them with water for 5–6 minutes.
Usage: Frequently drink it as a tea substitute.
Efficacy: It can dispel the toxicity of alcohol, and reduce its side effects.

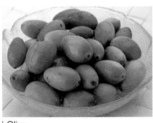

| Olive.

2. Olive tea
Ingredients: 30 g fresh olive.
Procedure: Simmer or soak the olives.
Usage: Drink it as a tea substitute.
Efficacy: It can dispel the effects of alcohol.

Dysentery and Bacterial Disease

As a kind of enteric infectious disease caused by shigella dysenteriae, dysentery is featured by acute diarrhea, stomachache and fever. Treating dysentery with tea has been a common therapy in China since ancient times. While dysentery is now relatively rare and would usually be treated by Western medicine, tea can also restrain typhoid bacillus and other bacterial diseases. It is believed that drinking a proper amount of tea can promote digestion and prevent communicable diseases of the gastrointestinal tract.

The effectual mechanism is primarily related to the antibacterial function of tea. This is mainly due to the effects of tea polyphenol, especially gallocatechin and flavone, which can help to stop diarrhea and protect the mucous membranes of the intestinal wall. In addition, when bacterioprotein meets tea polyphenols, they will cohere and lose their function. This bacteriostatic effect of green tea is better than that of black tea.

Flavanol compounds in tea can directly diminish inflammation, working against the inflammatory factor histamine, and can reduce permeability of blood capillaries. Tea also contains abundant nutrients needed by the human body such as vitamins C and B, which is of great benefit to overall health. Various kinds of tea are effective, although green tea is best.

1. Ginger and dark plum tea

Ingredients: 10 g ginger, 30 g dried dark plums, 6 g green tea leaves, brown sugar.

Procedure: Chop up ginger and plum, and infuse with boiling water. Soak for half an hour and add brown sugar.

Usage: Three times a day. Take it when it is warm.

Efficacy: It has the effects of removing internal heat to promote salivation, stopping dysentery (bacillary and amebic) and helping digestion, as well as warming the intestines and stomach.

2. Rice porridge tea

Ingredients: 10 g tea leaves, 50 g rice, white sugar.

Procedure: Simmer tea leaves in water for about 1,000 ml of extraction. Discard tea leaves, add rice and white sugar, and about 400 ml of water to make porridge.

Usage: Twice per day. Take it when it is warm.

Efficacy: It has the effects of tonifying the spleen and promoting diuresis, tonifying *qi* and refreshing oneself, as well as curing dysentery. It is taken for acute and chronic dysentery as well as enteritis.

3. Three-juice tea

Ingredients: 2.5 ml ginger juice, 5 ml honey, 10 ml radish juice, 15 g tea leaves.

Procedure: First simmer tea leaves for strong extraction. Add the ginger, radish and honey, and mix.

Usage: One dose per day. Take it when it is warm.

Efficacy: It has the effects of clearing internal heat, resolving dampness and stopping dysentery (taken for red-white dysentery).

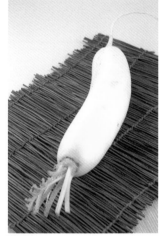

| Radish.

4. Tangerine peel and ginger tea

Ingredients: 10 g old tea leaves, 10 g tangerine peel, 7 g ginger.

Procedure: Simmer in water for 5–10 minutes.

Usage: Get the extraction and drink it as long as it is warm, whenever you like. Two to three doses per day.

Efficacy: It has the effects of clearing internal heat and promoting diuresis, regulating the functions of the intestines and stomach as well as the flow of vital energy. It is taken for hot dysentery, tenesmus (constant feeling of the need to defecate), and diarrhea and discharge.

5. Mung bean tea

Ingredients: Mung bean powder, tea leaves, white sugar.

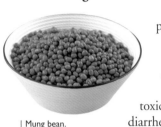

Procedure: Soak equal amounts of mung bean powder and tea leaves in boiling water, and then mix with sugar.

Usage: Taken it at a draught, meaning at one go relatively quickly.

Efficacy: It can clear away internal heat and toxic materials, regulate the middle *jiao* and stop diarrhea. It is taken for cholera, vomiting and diarrhea.

| Mung bean.

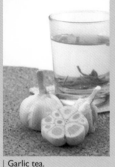

Additional Recipe for Chronic Dysentery—Garlic Tea

Ingredients: 60 g green tea leaves (longjing tea is the most suitable), 1 piece garlic (unpeeled whole garlic).

Procedure: First peel off the skin of the garlic, and then smash it into mash. Soak it with tea leaves in boiling water.

Usage: Twice or three times per day. Usually, the treatment lasts for 4–5 days.

Efficacy: It is taken for chronic dysentery.

| Garlic tea.

Gastroenteritis

Enteritis is a kind of intestinal inflammation caused by bacteria, with the main symptom being diarrhea. The therapy is similar to that for dysentery, but the ailment is less serious without infectivity. Enteritis can be divided into two types: acute and chronic, with the former having gastritis at the same time, thus being called acute gastroenteritis.

It usually takes only a short time to cure acute enteritis with tea therapy, with all symptoms, including bowel movements, likely to return to normal within one or two days.

1. Dried ginger green tea
Ingredients: 3 g green tea leaves, 3 g dried ginger.
Procedure: Put into a cup and infuse with boiling water. Cover the cup and soak for 10 minutes.
Usage: Frequently drink it as a tea substitute.
Efficacy: It is taken for acute gastroenteritis.

2. Powdered dried ginger green tea
Ingredients: 60 g green tea leaves, 30 g dried ginger.
Procedure: Grind them into fine powder.
Usage: Use 3 g of the powder with boiling water, 2–3 times per day.
Efficacy: It is taken for acute gastroenteritis.

3. Baked ginger rice tea
Ingredients: 15 g tea leaves, 3 g baked ginger, 30 g rice.
Procedure: Simmer with water.
Usage: Drink it as a tea substitute.
Efficacy: It is especially effective for those with chronic diarrhea and cold-deficiency in the spleen and stomach.

4. Plantain seed tea
Ingredients: 10 g fried plantain seeds, 3 g black tea leaves.
Procedure: Infuse with boiling water for strong extraction and cover for 10 minutes. Or simmer these two things for strong extraction.
Usage: Separate into two doses, and take when warm, 1–2 doses per day.
Efficacy: It is taken for insufficiency of the spleen and watery diarrhea.

5. Pilose asiabell and rice tea
Ingredients: 25 g root of pilose asiabell, 50 g rice (fried until yellow and dried).
Procedure: Simmer with 4 cups of water until there are 2 cups of extraction.
Usage: Drink it as a tea substitute when warm, finishing the dose within one day. Take once every two days continuously.
Efficacy: It is taken for insufficiency of the spleen and diarrhea as well as chronic gastritis.

Chronic Hepatitis and Cirrhosis

As we have seen, tea contains such components as caffeine, theophylline, tannin, gallotannic acid, protein, vitamins and microelements, and it has the effects of clearing heat, helping digestion and promoting diuresis.

Special properties of green tea include promoting blood circulation to remove blood stasis as anticoagulation, preventing blood platelets from adhering and gathering, and lessening the decrease of white blood cells. It assists in treating those with chronic hepatitis and blood stasis characterized by restlessness and heat in the chest and the center of the palms and soles, bitter taste in the mouth and dry throat, and red, bleeding and swollen gums.

Drinking tea, especially green tea, is beneficial to physical and psychological health, but no matter the condition, it is important to drink the proper amount at the proper time. The taste of single green tea is best after it is soaked in cold (pre-boiled) water for 45 minutes before preparing.

1. Chinese lobelia combination tea

Ingredients: 600 g herb of Chinese lobelia, 300 g seedling of capillary wormwood, 800 g rhizome of lalang grass.

Procedure: Grind into rough powder. For one dose, use 50–70 g of the powder. Put in a vacuum flask, infuse with boiling water and soak for 15 minutes.

Usage: Drink it as a tea substitute, once per day.

Efficacy: It has the effects of clearing away internal heat and toxic materials, promoting diuresis and getting rid of jaundice. It is taken for a variety of symptoms and conditions, including jaundice hepatitis, fever with aversion to cold, poor appetite, lassitude, weakness all over the body, distinct yellow complexion, swelling pain in hepatic region, dry mouth, dark urine, reddened tongue or yellow and greasy coating on the tongue, and thready pulse.

2. Giant knotweed combination tea

Ingredients: 600 g rhizome of giant knotweed, 600 g seedling of capillary wormwood, 600 g indigowoad root , 600 g dandelion, 200 g tangerine peel.

Procedure: Grind them together into powder. For one dose, use 60–90 g of powder and put into a vacuum flask. Infuse with a proper amount of boiling water, and cover for 15–20 minutes.

Usage: Drink it as a tea substitute once daily, at any time of day.

Efficacy: It has the effects of clearing away internal heat and toxic substances, and relieving jaundice. It is mainly taken for acute viral hepatitis, with the symptoms being poor appetite and a particular disgust for greasy or oily foods, weakness, nausea, pain in the hepatic region, enlargement of the liver or spleen, abdominal distension, and deficiencies indicated by the liver function test.

3. Carp and black tea

Ingredients: 20 g black tea leaves, 1 piece carp.

Procedure: Boil a carp with black tea for extraction. The carp can also be eaten. Or you can add 10 g of turmeric rhizome (curcuma longa) and 15 g wolfberries.

Usage: Take it without salt.

Efficacy: It is mainly taken for ascites (accumulation of fluid in abdominal cavity) caused by hepatitis.

4. Tumeric liver-purifying tea

Ingredients: 10 g turmeric rhizome, 5 g honey-fried licorice root, 2 g green tea leaves, 25 g honey.

Procedure: Add 1,000 ml of water and boil for 10 minutes.

Usage: Finish the dose within one day. Take it frequently whenever you like.

Efficacy: It can soothe liver-*qi* stagnation, promote diuresis and rid stagnation. It is taken for hepatitis, cirrhosis and fatty liver.

5. Plum tea

Ingredients: 100–150 g fresh plums, 2 g green tea leaves, 25 g honey.

Procedure: Slice the fresh plums, add 320 ml of water and boil for 3 minutes. Then add tea leaves and honey, and after bringing to a boil again, drink the extraction.

Usage: One dose per day, split into three portions, to take in the morning, at noon and in the evening, respectively.

Efficacy: It has the effects of clearing internal heat and promoting diuresis, nourishing the liver and eliminating stagnation. It is taken for cirrhosis and ascites.

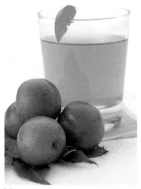

| Plum tea.

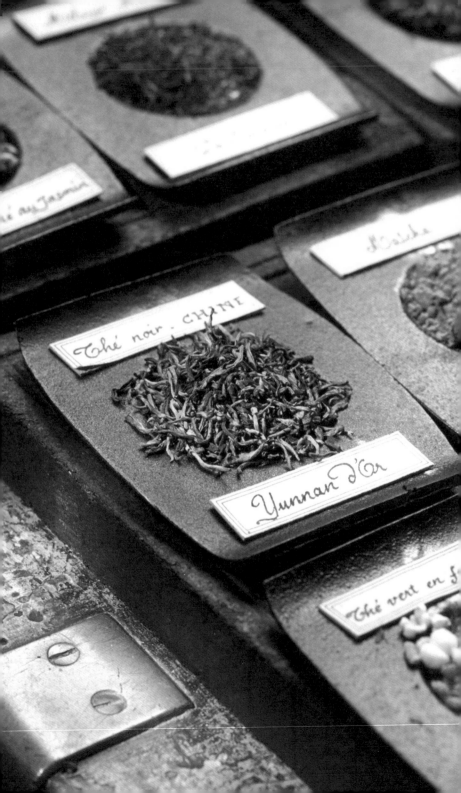

Chapter 6
Resisting Diseases of
the Respiratory System

The respiratory system connects directly to the external environment, and the lung is also the only organ receiving all the blood transported from the heart, with a large volume of blood flow. This means that noxious gas, dust and pathogenic microorganisms from the outside as well as allergens and pathogenic factors in the blood can easily invade the lung and cause disease.

In the past, the most common diseases of the respiratory system were infectious diseases, especially bacterial pneumonia and tuberculosis. With the increasingly common application of antibiotics, most of these have been effectively controlled. Other factors have become more prevalent, however. Due to atmospheric pollution, smoking and other factors, the morbidity and fatality rates of chronic obstructive pulmonary disease, lung cancer, occupational lung disease, and chronic pulmonary heart disease, among others, continue to grow, and deserve sufficient attention.

| As there is a wide variety of tea, one should choose a suitable kind according to one's physique and constitution to keep the respiratory system healthy.

Common Cold

Common cold is a disease of acute inflammation in the nose and throat caused by virus or bacteria. It is most usual in winter and spring, and shows strong infectivity. While the cause is viral or bacterial, getting wet and/or chilled and being over-tired can be contributing factors.

The disease usually comes on very quickly with such symptoms as nasal obstruction, runny nose, sneezing, throat itch or pain, and cough. In light cases, patients have a low-grade fever and are intolerant of cold; as for serious cases, patients have fever, headache, muscular stiffness, weakness and hoarseness, among other symptoms.

Since ancient times, people have treated the common cold with tea. For example, the Szechwan lovage mixture from the classic text *Prescriptions of Peaceful Benevolent Dispensary* is still extensively applied to cure common cold. Many components in tea play a role. Caffeine and theophylline can promote diuresis and clear internal heat, tea polyphenol can inhibit and kill bacteria, catechin can treat headache, and Vitamin C can strengthen the constitution and fight against infection.

1. Szechwan lovage mixture

Ingredients: 6 g rhizome of Szechwan lovage, 3 g herb of Manchurian wildginger, 6 g root of dahuriae angelica, 6 g root of incised notopterygium, 3 g licorice root, 6 g herb of fineleaf schizonepeta, 6 g root of divaricate saposhnikovia, 3 g mint, 3 g tea leaves.

Procedure: Grind everything except tea leaves into fine powder.

Usage: Take the powder with tea.

Efficacy: It evacuates wind-evil and stops headache. It is mainly taken for exogenous pathogenic wind, migraine or head pain, intolerance of cold, fever, dizziness, desire to vomit, nasal obstruction, and runny nose. This prescription enjoys a high reputation, since it was already widely applied in the Song dynasty more than 1,000 years ago.

2. Black tea therapy

Ingredients: 5 g black tea leaves, yellow rice wine.

Procedure: Boil or soak black tea leaves for 5 minutes, get the extraction and add some yellow rice wine.

Usage: One to two doses per day, taking half of the above recipe as a dose.

Efficacy: It is taken for common cold with headache, dizziness, sensation of chill and ache in arms and legs.

3. Wushen tea

Ingredients: 10 g herb of fineleaf schizonepeta, 10 g purple perilla leaves, 10 g ginger, 6 g tea leaves, 30 g brown sugar.

Procedure: Decoct all of the above except for brown sugar over low flame for 10–15 minutes, and then add brown sugar, stirring until it dissolves.

Usage: Drink it as a tea substitute.

Efficacy: It has the effects of diffusing wind-cold, dispelling wind and relieving pain. It is taken for common cold due to wind-cold, intolerance of cold, body pain and absence or reduction of sweating.

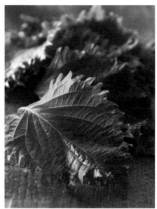

| Purple perilla leaf.

4. Flower mint tea

Ingredients: 10 g tea leaves, 3 g rose buds, 5 g mint, 5 g chrysanthemum.

Procedure: Infuse with 200 ml of boiling water.

Usage: After soaking for 5 minutes, drink when warm. The mixture can be reused by adding additional boiling water 1–3 times per day.

Efficacy: With its pungent flavor and cool property, it has the effects of relieving exterior syndrome, clearing internal heat and quenching one's thirst. It is taken for headache due to pathogenic wind-heat, cough and dry mouth.

5. Magnolia flower tea

Ingredients: 10 g tea leaves, 5 g magnolia flower buds, 5 g rhizome of Szechwan lovage, 3 g mint.

Procedure: Infuse with 200 ml of boiling water.

Usage: Take it at a draught.

Efficacy: It can relieve superficial syndrome with its pungent and warm nature. It helps to relieve allergic sinusitis, common cold, nasal obstruction and cough.

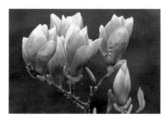

| Magnolia flower.

6. Szechwan lovage sugar tea

Ingredients: 6 g rhizome of Szechwan lovage, 6 g green tea leaves, brown sugar.

Procedure: Decoct these three things with one and a half cups of water till there is only one cup of extraction. Drink the tea only.

Usage: Drink it as a tea substitute.

Efficacy: It can dispel the wind and cold in the body. It is taken for headache and pain in the back caused by external cold, aversion to wind and intolerance of cold.

7. Purple perilla combination tea

Ingredients: 4.5 g purple perilla leaves, 4.5 g wrinkled gianthyssop, 4.5 g mint, 4.5 g herb of fineleaf schizonepeta, 5 g tea leaves.

Procedure: Grind into rough powder and infuse with boiling water.

Usage: Drink it as a tea substitute.

Efficacy: It can dispel wind and relieve exterior syndrome, as well as prevent and treat common cold.

8. Prune black tea

Ingredients: 1 prune (any kind is acceptable), one big spoonful of black tea leaves.

Procedure: First get rid of the kernel and chop the prune. Mix it with black tea leaves, and infuse with 200 ml of boiling water for 10 minutes.

Usage: Two doses per day. Take it when it is warm at any time of day.

Efficacy: It has the effects of dispelling cold, stopping coughing and stimulating the appetite. It is taken for preventing common cold and coughing in winter. It is especially suitable for children.

9. Mint tea

Ingredients: 2 g mint, 5 g tea leaves.

Procedure: Soak in boiling water and add sugar.

Usage: Frequently drink it as a tea substitute.

Efficacy: It can relieve exterior syndrome with its pungent flavor and cool property. It is taken for external infection of wind-heat, headache, conjunctival congestion, dyspepsia and abdominal distention.

10. Purple perilla and notopterygium tea

Ingredients: 9 g purple perilla leaves, 9 g root of incised notopterygium, 9 g tea leaves.

Procedure: Grind into rough powder and infuse with boiling water.

Usage: One dose per day. Take it when it is warm at any time.

Efficacy: It can relieve superficial syndrome with its pungent and warm nature. It is taken for common cold due to wind-cold, fever with aversion to cold, lack of normal sweating, and ache in arms and legs.

11. Spiced walnut tea

Ingredients: 25 g walnut, 25 g white scallion, 25 g ginger, 15 g tea leaves.

Procedure: Mash walnut, white scallion and ginger, making a paste with tea leaves. Add one and a half cups of water for decoction, and drink the tea only.

Usage: One dose per day. Take it at a draught, warm. Lie in bed covered with quilt and wait until you are sweating. Make sure to stay out of the wind.

Efficacy: It can relieve exterior syndrome and dispel cold, induce sweating and bring down a fever. It is taken for common cold, fever, headache, body pain and lack of sweating.

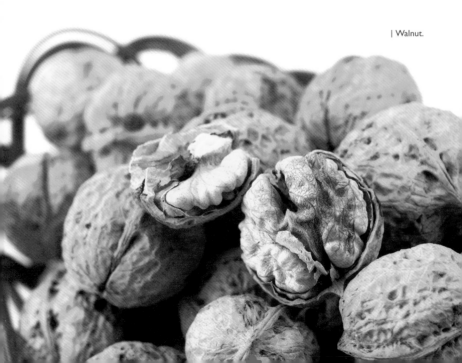

| Walnut.

12. Mint and reed rhizome tea

Ingredients: 10 g fresh mint, 60 g fresh reed rhizome.

Procedure: Clean and chop, then put in a vacuum flask and infuse with boiling water.

Usage: Frequently drink it as a tea substitute.

Efficacy: It has the effects of dispersing exterior evil, opening inhibited lung-energy and relieving sore throat. It is mainly taken for summer dryness and autumn heat, sore throat caused by sleeping in the open at night, and for wind, dry cough, thirst, intolerance of cold, and to induce sweating. It mustn't be taken by those with summer heat and damp, fever, diarrhea, or a thick and greasy coating on the tongue.

13. Tea for flu

Ingredients: 30 g cyrtomium rhizome, 30 g indigowoad root, 15 g licorice root.

Procedure: Soak in boiling water.

Usage: Drink it as a tea substitute. One dose per day, taken whenever you like.

Efficacy: It can dispel wind, clear internal heat and relieve sore throat. It is taken for the flu.

Cough and Asthma

A cough is caused by an impulse transmitted to the brain after the respiratory tract is subject to stimulation by inflammation, foreign matters or other factors. It is a natural way for the body to protect itself by discharging secretion or foreign matters, and clearing the respiratory tract. Therefore coughing is usually a beneficial action. Under normal conditions, for light and infrequent coughing, the situation can be relieved as long as sputum or other obstructions are discharged and there is no need to take antitussive drugs.

However, drastic dry cough without phlegm, or frequent intense cough with phlegm, can bring pain and interfere with sleep, increase the patient's physical exhaustion, and even aggravate a condition and cause other complications. Consequently, it is more harmful.

Several components in tea are effective against coughing and asthma. It is known that theophylline and caffeine can relax smooth muscle and relieve bronchial spasms. Tea polyphenol can control and kill bacteria as well as diminish inflammation, while aromatic substances in tea can eliminate phlegm.

1. Tangerine tea
Ingredients: 3–6 g of the orange part of tangerine peel, 4.5 g green tea leaves.

Procedure: Soak them in boiling water, and then steam this mixture for 20 minutes.

Usage: One dose per day. Take it frequently at any time of day.

Efficacy: It can moisten the lung and dissolve phlegm, regulate the flow of vital energy, and relieve a cough. It is taken for cough with excessive phlegm, or for sticky phlegm that is hard to expectorate.

2. White fungus tea
Ingredients: 20 g white fungus, 5 g tea leaves, 20 g rock candy (or large sugar crystals).

Procedure: First stew white fungus with rock candy, and soak tea leaves in boiling water for 5 minutes. Take the tea extraction and put it in the white fungus liquid.

Usage: One dose per day. Take it frequently whenever you like.

Efficacy: It can nourish *yin*, reduce internal heat, moisten lungs to arrest cough, and cure deficiency of *yin*, cough, tuberculosis and low-grade fever.

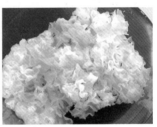
| White fungus tea.

3. Asthma-relieving tea
Ingredients: 3 g ephedra, 4.5 g bark of Chinese corktree, 15 pieces of ginkgo nut (smashed), 6 g tea leaves, 30 g white sugar.

Procedure: Put the first four things in water, and decoct them for extraction. Then add white sugar.

Usage: The above creates one daily dose, which should be separated into two portions to be taken at different times.

Efficacy: It is taken for asthma, when an attack occurs and leads to difficult breathing. It has the effects of opening the inhibited lung-energy, purifying and descending *qi*, relieving asthma and stopping cough.

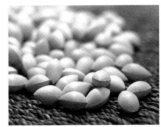
| Gingko nut.

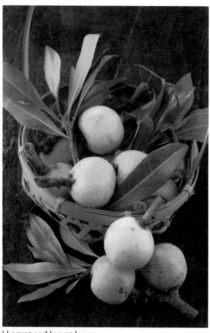

| Loquat and loquat leaves.

4. Loquat-leaf tea

Ingredients: 30 g fresh loquat leaves, 15 g herb of common lophatherum.

Procedure: Brush away the tomentum (or small "hairs") on the fresh loquat leaves, and wash both the loquat leaves and common lophatherum. Chop and put in a vacuum flask. Infuse with boiling water and cover for 15 minutes. Add some white sugar or rock candy if desired.

Usage: Frequently drink it as a tea substitute. One dose per day.

Efficacy: It can clear away lung-heat and depress *qi*, relieve cough and reduce sputum. It is mainly taken for cough with lung heat, dry throat and hoarseness. It mustn't be taken by patients with cough due to wind-cold evil.

5. Cough-relieving tea

Ingredients: 9 g root of pilose asiabell, 6 g purple perilla seeds, 6 g prepared pinellia rhizome, 6 g root of baikal skullcap, 4 g honey-fried licorice root.

Procedure: Grind all of the above into a rough powder and pack in a gauze bundle or filter paper. Put the bundle in a vacuum flask and infuse with boiling water. Cover for 15 minutes, then drink.

Usage: Frequently drink it as a tea substitute. One dose per day.

Efficacy: It has the function of resolving sputum and relieving asthma, and tonifying *qi* and lungs. It is mainly taken for chronic bronchitis, repeated cough with excessive phlegm, stuffy feeling in the chest, shortness of breath, inability to cough up sputum, and body fatigue and weakness.

Sphagitis

Sphagitis is an inflammation of the laryngopharynx and oropharynx in the upper throat, which is mainly caused by virus and bacterial infection. It may be chronic or acute. Prevention methods include:

- avoiding long-term exposure to dust, gas, chlorine, and ammonia;
- avoiding wearing down the body, including overuse of voice, working and exercising too hard, having insufficient sleep or bad sleep habits, or getting a chill;
- having a healthy, fresh diet, including foods with high water content such as radish, pears, waternut corms and fresh reed rhizome, and drinking sufficient water;
- taking less pungent and warm-dry food cooked in the way of stir-frying or frying, e.g. dried ginger, spice pepper and pepper, etc.;
- quitting smoking and drinking alcohol;
- keeping bowels functioning well to discharge deficiency-oriented heat;
- actively treating rhinitis and chronic tonsillitis to lessen irritation of the throat;
- preventing and curing such chronic diseases as anemia, constipation, chronic inflammation of the lower respiratory tract, and cardiovascular diseases, to improve blood stasis in the throat area and effectively prevent

| Chrysanthemum.

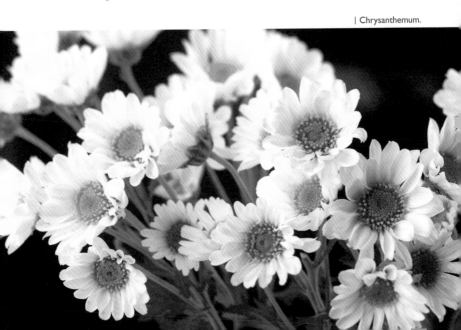

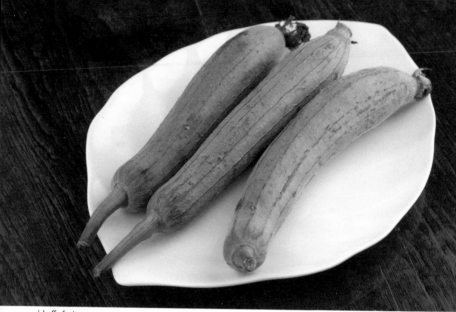

| Luffa fruit.

the disease from secondary onset.

Tea has certain preventative and therapeutic effects for acute and chronic sphagitis, as well as voice hoarseness and laryngitis due to repeated cough or other factors.

1. Chrysanthemum tea

Ingredients: 30 g fresh tea leaves, 30 g fresh chrysanthemum.

Ingredients: Mash up tea leaves and chrysanthemum for extraction, and mix the extraction with 30–60 ml of cold water that was previously boiled.

Usage: One dose per day, taken cold at any time you like.

Efficacy: It has the effects of clearing internal heat to reduce swelling, relieving sore throat and stopping pain. It is taken for acute and chronic sphagitis, sore throat, itchiness and discomfort in the throat as well as throat diseases.

2. Luffa fruit tea

Ingredients: 200 g luffa fruit (cut into slices), 5 g tea leaves, 2 g salt.

Procedure: First boil the luffa fruit with salt. Soak tea leaves separately in boiling water for 5 minutes. Then add the tea extraction to the luffa fruit liquid.

Usage: One dose per day. Take it whenever you like.

Efficacy: It has the effects of clearing internal heat and toxic materials, relieving cough and reducing sputum, and relieving sore throat. It is taken for acute and chronic sphagitis, itchiness and discomfort in the throat, tonsillitis and bronchitis, as well as cough.

3. Cortex albziae flower green tea

Ingredients: 3 g green tea leaves, 3 g cortex albziae flowers, 2 boat-fruited sterculia seeds, rock candy.

Procedure: Infuse with boiling water.

Usage: Drink it as a tea substitute.

Efficacy: It has the effect of clearing lung-heat and moistening dryness. It is taken for laryngitis and hoarseness.

4. Olive, bamboo-leaf and plum tea

Ingredients: 5 pieces salted olives, 5 g bamboo leaves, 2 dried dark plums, 5 g green tea leaves, 10 g white sugar.

Procedure: Decoct with water for extraction, simmering to make one cup of extraction.

Usage: Two doses per day. Take when it is warm.

Efficacy: It has the effects of clearing lung-heat and relieving throat dryness. It is taken for loss of voice, and both acute and chronic sphagitis, caused by repeated cough and overuse.

5. Momordica fruit and mint tea

Ingredients: 30 g momordica fruit, 10 g mint, 5 g olives (you may use fresh or dried, but the fresh one is of better therapeutic effect), 3 g licorice root.

Procedure: First cut momordica fruit into thin slices. Mince the mint leaf and mash the olives. Simmer them with licorice root in a pot for extraction.

Usage: Drink it as a tea substitute.

Efficacy: It has the effects of promoting production of body fluid and moistening dryness, relieving sore throat and dry throat. It works well for sphagitis, loss of voice, summer heat and excessive thirst, pyrophlegm and cough, and scanty dark urine.

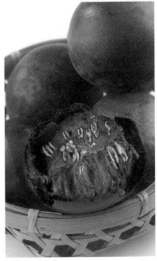

| Momordica fruit.

6. Double-flower tea

Ingredients: 10 g chrysanthemum, 10 g honeysuckle, 6 g licorice root, 6 g boat-fruited sterculia seeds.

Procedure: Put in a vacuum flask and infuse with boiling water.

Usage: Frequently drink it as a tea substitute. One dose per day.

Efficacy: It has the effects of dispelling wind and heat, relieving internal heat or fever, and clearing the voice. It is mainly taken for acute pharyngitis, tonsillitis, sore throat, voice hoarseness, and dry cough with no phlegm.

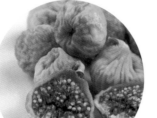

| Fig.

7. Momordica fruit and fig tea

Ingredients: 20 g momordica fruit, 20 g fig.

Procedure: Cut both into slices and simmer them in boiling water for 15 minutes.

Usage: Drink it as a tea substitute.

Efficacy: It has the effects of removing internal heat from the lungs to relieve cough as well as relaxing the bowels. As it can protect one's voice, it is good for those who speak a great deal as part of their professions, such as teachers and actors, to take it often. It is of comparatively good therapeutic effect for voice hoarseness due to lungs attacked by wind-heat.

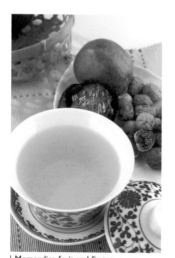

| Momordica fruit and fig tea.

8. Root tea

Ingredients: 6 g mint, 9 g root of four-leaf ladybell, 9 g stemona root, 4 g licorice root.

Procedure: First put the mint into a vacuum flask. Decoct the roots of ladybell, stemona and licorice with fresh water for 15 minutes. When boiling, pour the extraction in the flask. Cover it for 10 minutes.

Usage: Frequently drink it as a tea substitute.

Efficacy: It has the effects of opening inhibited lung-energy with its pungent flavor and cool property, moistening dryness and relieving cough. It is mainly taken for cool-dryness in autumn, dry cough with little or no phlegm, dry itch and discomfort in throat, and by people who are prone to feeling cold. It mustn't be taken by those with cough due to wind-cold evil or that with a great deal of white expectoration.

9. Osmanthus flower tea
Ingredients: 2 g tea leaves, 1 g osmanthus flowers.
Procedure: Soak tea leaves and osmanthus flowers in boiling water for 6 minutes.
Usage: One cup in the morning and one cup in the evening.
Efficacy: It should be taken by those with dry skin and hoarse voice.

Sinusitis

Sinusitis refers to a suppurative (or discharge-causing) inflammation due to infection of the mucous membrane of the nasal sinuses. There are acute and chronic cases, and this kind of disease can be aggravated by cold and decreased immunity of the body. Other nasal diseases, swimming and diving, and rapid change of air pressure (for example, when flying or diving) can also lead to the onset of this disease.

1. Siberian cocklebur combination tea
Ingredients: 12 g fruit of Siberian cocklebur, 9 g magnolia flower buds, 9 g root of dahuriae angelica, 4.5 g mint, 3 pieces white scallion, 2 g tea leaves.
Procedure: Grind the herbs into powder and infuse it with boiling water for 10 minutes.
Usage: One dose per day. Take it frequently whenever you like.
Efficacy: It has the effects of dispelling wind, inducing perspiration, and easing breathing through nose. It is taken for acute sinusitis and wind-cold exterior syndrome, fever with aversion to cold, and nasal obstruction with a runny nose.

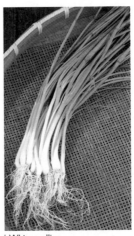
| White scallion.

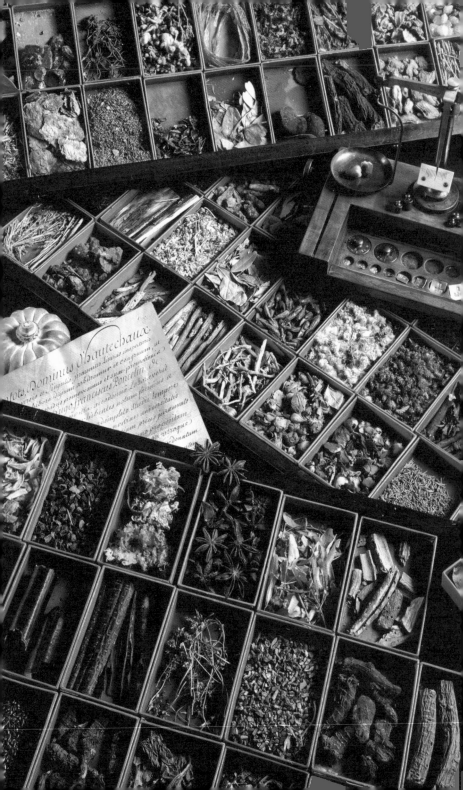

Chapter 7
Controlling Diseases of
Urinary System

There are various diseases related to the urinary system, many of which have symptoms and causes that can be treated with tea therapy. Since tea contains caffeine, theophylline and theobromine, it is helpful in promoting diuresis and enhancing kidney excretion, and it can be used for many ailments with difficult urination or nephritis.

As far as promoting diuresis is concerned, theophylline is better than caffeine, which is in turn better than theobromine. However clinical experiments show that even though the effect of promoting diuresis of theophylline is strong, that of theobromine is more enduring. The main way in which these components work is by restraining the re-absorption of kidney tubules, hence increasing the content of sodium and chloride ions in urine. Moreover since they can excite the vasomotor center, directly relax the vessels of kidney, and increase renal plasma flow, the filtration rate of the glomerulus is improved. This effect also helps to get rid of accumulations of extracellular water, as shown clinically.

Research shows that for patients with chronic renal failure, tea polyphenol can effectively decrease their procoagulant activity and reduce fibrinogen, hence improving microcirculation of the kidney,

| Chinese medicinal herbs, functioning as tea substitutes, are an important means of tea therapy, serving to promoting diuresis.

increasing the kidney blood flow volume and filtration rate of the glomerulus, and promoting excretion of metabolites. In addition, tea polyphenol can restrain the generation of oxygen radicals and improve organic oxidation resistance. This improves the activity of cellular superoxide dismutase and reduces the harm of radicals to the kidney.

Various kinds of tea can promote diuresis to a certain extent. However, patients with stones in the urinary system must drink tea with restraint, paying attention to the amount and methods. Patients with urethral calculus are advised to drink water instead of tea.

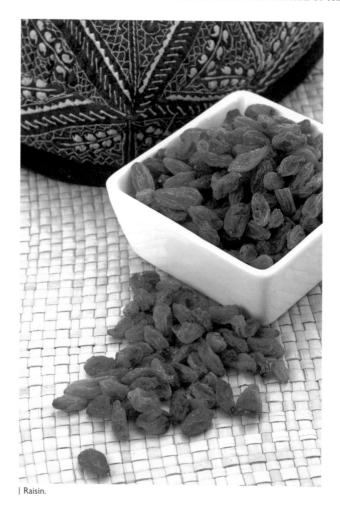

| Raisin.

1. Green tea with ephedra and raisins

Ingredients: 6 g stems of ephedra, 20 g raisins, 20 g green tea leaves, 20 g herb of tuberculate speranskia, 7 jujubes.

Procedure: Decoct with water.

Usage: The above makes one dose. Separate into two portions to take within one day. Continue for 4 days.

Efficacy: It has the effects of inducing perspiration, relieving exterior syndrome and promoting diuresis. It is taken for edema caused by acute nephritis.

2. Motherwort tea

Ingredients: 6–9 g motherwort fruit, 6–9 g tea leaves (use equal amounts).

Procedure: Add 600 ml of water and decoct till there is only 300 ml of extraction; or soak these two ingredients in boiling water for 20 minutes.

Usage: Two doses per day. Take on an empty stomach, finishing the entire dose at one go while hot.

Efficacy: It can clear internal heat and promote diuresis, and treat dark and turbid urine, as well as relieving urethral pain when urinating.

3. Lalang grass tea

Ingredients: 10 g lalang grass rhizome, 15 g tea leaves.

Procedure: Add water and boil for 15 minutes. Or cut the lalang grass rhizome into pieces and soak them with tea leaves in boiling water for 15 minutes.

Usage: One dose per day.

Efficacy: It has the effects of clearing internal heat and promoting diuresis, diminishing inflammation and detoxifying, and cooling blood and stopping bleeding. It is taken for acute and chronic nephritis, edema, acute infectious hepatitis and blood in the urine.

4. Astragalus root combination tea

Ingredients: 120 g astragalus root, 120 g shorthorned epimedium, 90 g rhizome of largehead atractylodes, 90 g root of divaricate saposhnikovia.

Procedure: Grind these four medicines into rough powder. Each time pack 30–40 g of the powder into a bundle. Put the bundle in a vacuum flask and infuse with boiling water, and then cover for 20 minutes.

Usage: Use 30–40 g (one bundle) each day, taking it at several different times during the day.

Efficacy: It has the effects of tonifying *qi* and the kidney as well as improving human immunity. It is mainly taken for latent nephritis, the syndromes of which are light red urine (or hematuria by microscopic examination), sleepiness, fatigue, spontaneous perspiration, intolerance of cold or liability to catch a cold, reduced appetite, edema, ache in waist and knees, dizziness and tinnitus, sallow complexion, light tongue nature (tongue is light or almost white in color), weak pulse, and kidney *yang* deficiency according to TCM diagnostic methods.

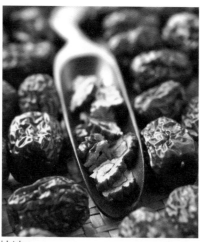

| Jujube.

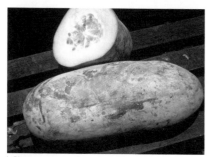

| Chinese waxgourd.

5. Snakehead combination tea

Ingredients: 1 piece fresh snakehead fish (weighing around 500 g), 200 g tea leaves, 500 g lalang grass rhizome, 500 g peel of Chinese waxgourd, 50 g ginger, 300 g jujubes, 250 g rock candy, 7 pieces white scallion.

Procedure: Decoct ingredients above with water till there is only about 1,000 ml of extraction. Put in fresh snakehead (cleaned), cook on low flame until done, and then add rock candy and white scallion.

Usage: Divide it into three parts to finish within a day. Drink the soup and eat the fish.

Efficacy: It has the effects of tonifying the spleen and kidney as well as inducing diuresis to reduce edema. It is taken for edema caused by nephritis.

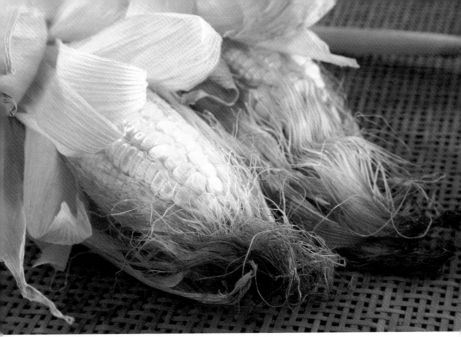

| Corn silk.

6. Corn silk tea

Ingredients: 30 g corn silk, 5 g tea leaves, 30 g lalang grass rhizome.

Procedure: Infuse with boiling water.

Usage: Drink as a tea substitute.

Efficacy: It can clear internal heat, promote diuresis and reduce blood pressure. It is taken for edema caused by nephritis complicated with hypertension.

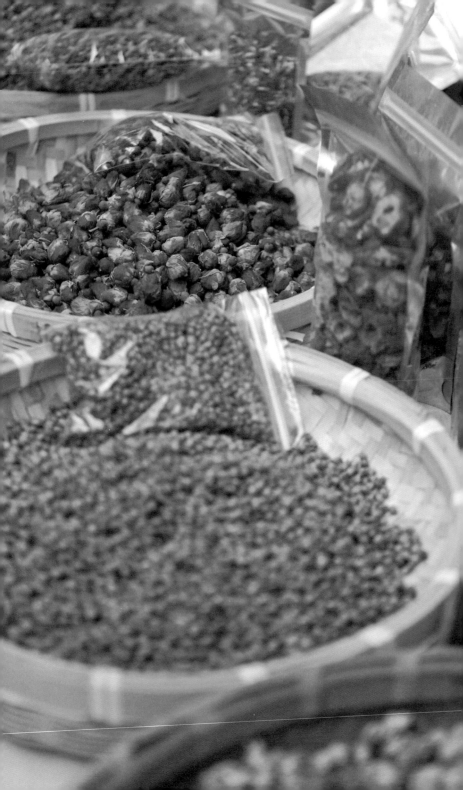

Chapter 8
Treating Gynecological Diseases

There are various kinds of gynecological diseases, which should be paid attention to and treated. If they are not, in many cases what was originally minor or latent might become serious and even lead to cancer. Tea can be used to treat gynecological diseases, due to the comprehensive effect of its many components.

| Flower tea is also an important variety of tea therapy. For instance, rose bud tea has certain effects on gynecological diseases.

1. Strong tea with brown sugar

Ingredients: Tea leaves and brown sugar.

Procedure: Decoct for one cup of strong tea.

Usage: Get the extraction and add brown sugar. Drink it after the brown sugar has dissolved completely. Take twice a day.

Efficacy: It has the effects of clearing internal heat and regulating menstruation. It is taken for premature menstruation and for menstruation with excessive bleeding.

2. Menstruation-regulating tea with Szechwan lovage

Ingredients: 3 g rhizome of Szechwan lovage, 6 g tea leaves.

Procedure: Decoct with water.

Usage: Drink it as a tea substitute, 1–2 doses per day.

Efficacy: It has the effects of invigorating the circulation of blood, removing stasis, promoting the circulation of *qi* and relieving pain. It is taken for irregular, painful or lack of menstruation; postpartum abdominal pain; head-wind and headache; and chest stuffiness and pains.

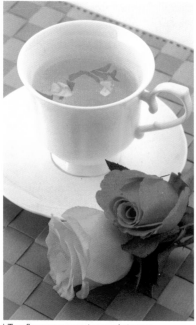

| Two-flower menstruation-regulating tea.

3. Two-flower menstruation-regulating tea

Ingredients: 9 g dried rose (or 18 g fresh), 9 g dried Chinese rose (or 18 g fresh), 3 g black tea leaves.

Procedure: Grind into rough powder. Infuse with boiling water and cover for 10 minutes.

Usage: Take when warm, at any time of day. It is better to take it before the menstrual period begins.

Efficacy: It has the effects of invigorating the circulation of blood, regulating menstruation and regulating *qi* to alleviate pain. It is taken for scanty or painful menstruation, abdominal distension and pain, menses with dark color or clots, and amenorrhea (lack of menstruation) caused by *qi*-stagnation and blood stasis.

4. Safflower tea with brown sugar
Ingredients: 5 g safflower, 5 g green tea leaves, 25 g brown sugar.

Procedure: To prepare safflower, douse it with vinegar, and fry over low flame until it is dry. Then soak these three medicines in 600 ml of water for 30 minutes.

Usage: This makes one daily dose, which should be split into four portions taken at 4-hour intervals.

Efficacy: It is taken for amenorrhea.

5. Jasmine tea
Ingredients: 1 g green tea leaves, 5 g jasmine.

Procedure: Decoct jasmine in 400 ml of water till it boils, and add green tea leaves after it has been boiling for 3 minutes.

Usage: One dose per day, split into 3 portions.

Efficacy: It is taken for excessive vaginal discharge (leukorrhea).

6. Purple perilla combination tea
Ingredients: 6 g purple perilla stems, 3 g tangerine peel, 2 slices ginger, 1 g black tea leaves.

Procedure: Cover ingredients in boiling water and soak for 10 minutes, or decoct them for 10 minutes.

Usage: One dose per day, split into 2–3 portions.

Efficacy: It has the effects of regulating the flow of vital energy and removing hiccups. It is useful in preventing miscarriage. It is taken for pernicious vomiting, nausea with vomiting, dizziness, and purging or immediate vomiting after eating food.

7. Hawthorn green tea
Ingredients: 2 g green tea leaves, 25 g Chinese hawthorn berry flakes.

Procedure: Add 400 ml of water and boil for 5 minutes.

Usage: One dose per day, split into 3 portions and taken warm. Boiled water can be added to mixture for use

| Chinese hawthorn berry flakes.

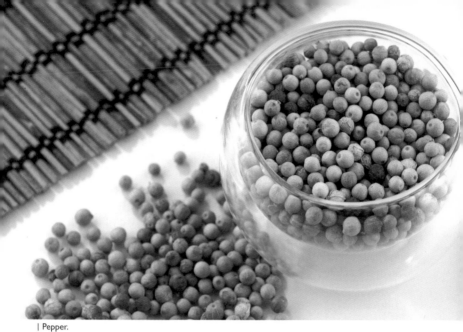

| Pepper.

several times.

Efficacy: It is taken for postpartum abdominal pain.

8. Brown sugar tea with pepper

Ingredients: 3 g tea leaves, 15 g brown sugar, 1.5 g pepper.

Procedure: Grind pepper into powder, and fry the brown sugar till it is scorched. Mix them with tea leaves and infuse with boiling water.

Usage: Drink it as a tea substitute. Or add 10 g motherwort herb and decoct them together. You may also add hot yellow rice wine.

Efficacy: It is taken for postpartum diarrhea and abdominal pain.

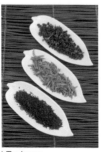

| Tea leaves.

9. Honey tea

Ingredients: 3 g tea leaves, 2 ml honey.

Procedure: Infuse with boiling water and wait for 5 minutes.

Usage: One to two doses per day, warm. Take one cup after meals.

Efficacy: It has the effects of relaxing bowels, tonifying lungs and relieving a cough. It is recommended that women take it for postpartum constipation, lung dryness and dry cough.

10. Corncob tea

Ingredients: 30 g corncob, sugar.

Procedure: Cut up the corncob, and decoct with water for extraction. Then add some sugar.

Usage: Drink it as a tea substitute.

Efficacy: It is taken for postpartum abnormal sweating due to general weakness, and night sweating.

11. Double-flower green tea

Ingredients: 10 g honeysuckle, 10 g wild chrysanthemum, 10 g green tea leaves.

Procedure: Decoct with water.

Usage: Drink it as a tea substitute. Take it every day for 5 days.

Efficacy: It has the effects of clearing or decreasing internal heat as well as dispersing toxins and swelling. It is taken for red and swollen nipples with pain and heat.

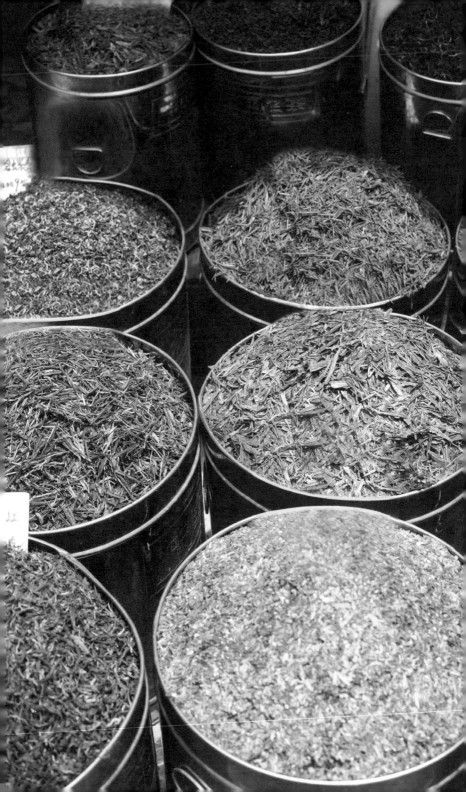

Chapter 9
Eye Care

Drinking tea helps protect and maintain healthy eyes, and its effect of improving eyesight was noted very early on and recorded in ancient books like *Gleaning Herbs*. It can be used in treating many common eye diseases including acute conjunctivitis and inflammation of the eyelid, as well as visual acuity issues, including nearsightedness, nyctalopia (night blindness) and cataract. Tea contains many kinds of nutritional components, especially vitamins, which are extremely important for nourishing the eyes.

| Thanks to its rich nutrient content, tea serves to improve eyesight.

Blurred Vision

Experiments have shown that the content of Vitamin C in the lens of the eye is much higher than in other tissues. That is to say, the demand for Vitamin C by the eye lens is higher, and if the intake is not sufficient, the lens will become turbid and affected by cataract. Tea has a high content of Vitamin C, so drinking tea can help to prevent cataracts.

The Vitamin B_1 contained in tea helps maintain the physiological functions of nerves, including the optic nerve. If one lacks this vitamin, one may develop optic neuritis, which will cause blurred vision and dry eyes.

Tea also contains a large amount of Vitamin B_2. The content is about five times higher than that in soybeans, twenty times higher than that in rice, and sixty times higher than that in fruit. It can nourish the epithelial tissues of the eyes and is indispensible to maintaining normal functions of the retina. Therefore, drinking tea can prevent and treat corneal opacity and inflammation (keratitis), dry eyes, photophobia or light-sensitivity and deterioration of eyesight due to the lack of Vitamin B_2.

1. Climbing groundsel tea
Ingredients: 30 g herb of climbing groundsel, 5 g licorice root.
Procedure: Infuse with boiling water.
Usage: Drink it as a tea substitute. Two doses per day.
Efficacy: It clears internal heat and toxic materials, helping to treat acute conjunctivitis; swollen sore throat; acute suppurative infection of the hair follicle, sebaceous gland and sudoriferous gland caused by bacteria; eczema; and dysentery.

Nyctalopia

The onset of nyctalopia (night blindness) is mainly related to the lack of Vitamin A. Even though dissociative Vitamin A hasn't been found in fresh tea leaves, abundant Provitamin A (i.e., carotene) has been found. In 100 g of dry tea leaves, the content of Vitamin A is about 16 mg in green tea leaves and 7–9 mg in black tea leaves.

After being absorbed by the body, carotene can turn into Vitamin A in the liver and small intestines, maintaining the normal function and state of epithelial tissues. Inside the retina, it also synthesizes with protein into rhodopsin, which is related to human scotopic vision, the vision of the eye under low light conditions.

Moreover, Vitamin A can maintain the integrity of the structure of epithelial tissues and their functions. Lack of this vitamin can affect the lacrimal gland epithelium, decreasing the secretion of tears and leading to xerophthalmia (abnormal dryness of the conjunctiva and cornea of the eyes). It can also cause the cornea and conjunctiva to be easily infected and form discharge, and even lead to serious diseases such as keratomalacia and corneal perforation.

As a result, drinking green tea rich in Vitamin A is of vital importance in preventing nyctalopia, xerophthalmia and keratitis, especially for those who often watch television. Many kinds of tea have this kind of curative effect but green tea is especially good in this aspect.

1. Wolfberry and chrysanthemum green tea
Ingredients: 10 g wolfberries, 10 g chrysanthemum, 3 g green tea leaves.

Procedure: Infuse with boiling water and cover for 10 minutes.

Usage: One dose per day. Drink it frequently.

Efficacy: It has the effects of nourishing the liver and kidneys, dispelling wind and improving eyesight. It is effective for treating deterioration of eyesight, dizziness, night blindness and juvenile nearsightedness.

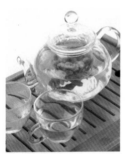
| Wolfberry and chrysanthemum green tea.

2. Mulberry leaf tea for conjunctivitis
Ingredients: 6 g mulberry leaves, 6 g honeysuckle, 6 g plantain herb.

Procedure: Grind these medicines into rough powder and infuse with boiling water.

Usage: Drink it as a tea substitute. One dose per day.

Efficacy: It is taken for acute conjunctivitis.

3. Cassia seed vision-improving tea
Ingredients: 20 g cassia seeds.

Procedure: Infuse with boiling water for 20 minutes.

Usage: Drink it as a tea substitute.

Efficacy: It has the effects of clearing the liver and improving vision. It can prevent and treat various kinds of wind-heat and pinkeye, e.g. acute conjunctivitis, hot eyes and soreness. It is also effective for optic atrophy and nyctalopia.

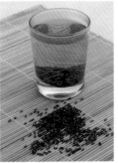
| Cassia seed vision-improving tea.

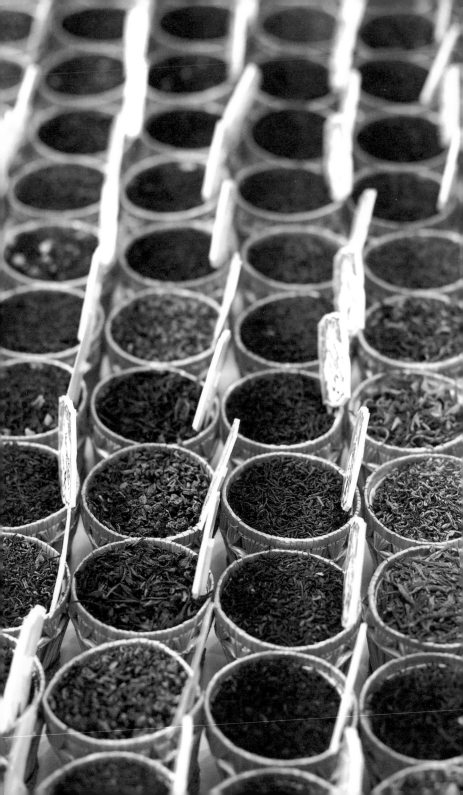

Chapter 10
Oral Health

A Dream of Red Mansions, a treasure of ancient Chinese literature, often mentions that members of the Jia family had the habit of using tea for dental care. For example, in Chapter 54 it says that during the Lantern Festival, the family enjoyed themselves until after midnight, eating jujube rice porridge and various kinds of exquisite pickled vegetables, and then "after drinking tea to rinse their mouths, they were dispersed." So the use of tea in maintaining oral health clearly has a long history in China.

| Fragrant tea not only has a curative effect on physical ailments, but also can dispel odors.

Tooth Decay and Cavities

As proven by modern scientific research, drinking tea can prevent tooth decay and strengthen teeth. These effects are mainly related to components, such as fluorine and tea polyphenol, contained in tea.

Tea trees are rich in fluorine, with the content ten times, or in some cases, even several hundred times, higher than that in ordinary plants. A dental researcher in America has studied tea leaves from different places in the world, and found that among 55 kinds of tea leaves, the fluorine content in oolong tea and green tea from China was the highest, and the effect of preventing tooth decay was the best.

The fluorine ion can prevent tooth decay and strengthen bones. In 100 g of tea leaves, there is about 10–15 mg of fluorine, and 80% of the fluorine can dissolve in the extraction. That means that by drinking the extraction from 10 g of tea leaves every day, one can get 1 mg of fluorine, which is beneficial to teeth.

Apart from fluorine's effect, the polyphenols in tea also have an important function in preventing tooth decay. A concentration of 1–2 mg/ml of tea polyphenol can restrain such decay-promoting bacteria as streptococcus mutans and lactobacillus.

The effectiveness of the components in tea relates to factors such as the age and quality of tea leaves. The content of fluorine in rough and old tea leaves is higher than those in tea shoots and tender tea leaves, and that in low-grade tea is higher than that in high-grade tea. Therefore, in terms of the effect of preventing tooth decay, it is better to take low-grade tea, which is also more economical.

1. Tea for strengthening teeth
Ingredients: 1–3 g tea leaves.
Procedure: Infuse with boiling water.
Usage: One to two cups a day. Drink the tea and rinse the mouth with tea.
Efficacy: It can remove contaminants, clean teeth and prevent tooth decay.

2. Tea for protecting teeth
Ingredients: 30 g black tea leaves.
Procedure: Add 500–1,000 ml of water and simmer till there is

only 250–500 ml of extraction. Drink the tea only.

Usage: One to three times per day. First, rinse the mouth with the tea and then drink it.

Efficacy: It has the effects of clearing internal heat, removing contaminants and protecting teeth. It is taken for periodontitis and sensitive teeth.

3. Manchurian wildginger and licorice tea

Ingredients: 4 g herb of Manchurian wildginger, 10 g honey-fried licorice root, 1 g green tea leaves.

Procedure: Add 400–500 ml of water, boil 5 minutes and then add 1 g of green tea leaves.

Usage: One dose per day, split into three portions. Take it after meals.

Efficacy: It works against tooth decay.

Halitosis

Drinking tea can increase the flow of liquid in the mouth and maintain oral hygiene. Tea components such as saccharides and pectin will have chemical reactions when encountering saliva, thus moistening the mouth and improving its self-cleaning capability.

1.Breath-freshening osmanthus tea

Ingredients: 3 g osmanthus flowers, 1 g black tea leaves.

Procedure: Put osmanthus flowers in 150 ml of water, bring to boil and then add black tea leaves.

Usage: One dose per day. Take it slowly.

Efficacy: It can help treat halitosis.

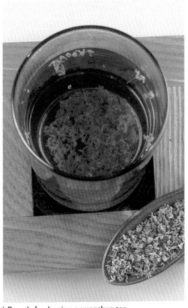

| Breath-freshening osmanthus tea.

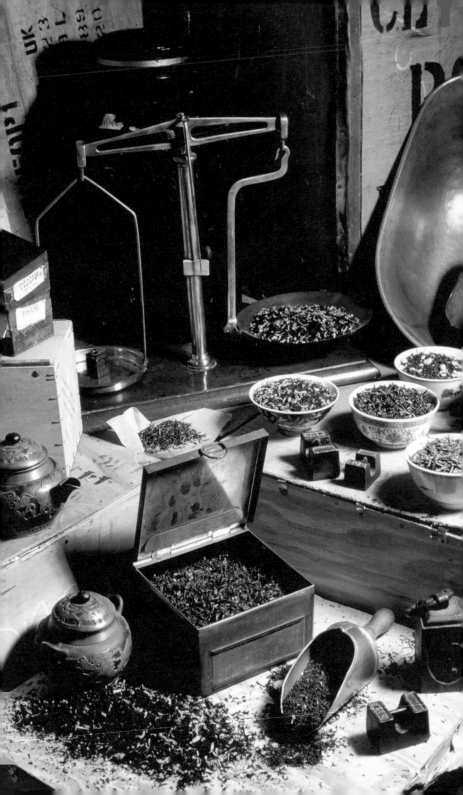

Chapter 11
Controlling Diabetes

Diabetes is a syndrome characterized by continuous hyperglycemia or excess blood glucose levels. There are various causes of insulin deficiency or lack of a normal response to insulin, leading to abnormal sugar, protein and fat metabolism in the human body, thus resulting in diabetes.

If diabetes is not controlled, certain metabolic disorders will become more serious, leading to chronic complications in tissues and organs such as the eyes, kidneys, nerves, vessels and heart. The final results may be blindness, gangrene of lower limbs, uremia, cerebral apoplexy or myocardial infarction, and even fatality.

The tea polyphenol and Vitamin C contained in tea can maintain normal strength and permeability of blood capillaries. This means that patients with diabetes who have frail blood capillaries can restore their normal functions through drinking tea.

What's more important is that tea also contains ingredients that prevent and treat abnormal sugar metabolism. Methyl salicylate in the aromatic substances of tea can improve the content of hepatic glycogen in the liver and decrease blood sugar. Vitamin B1 in tea is the constitutive substance of cocarboxylase and an indispensible coenzyme promoting glycometabolism, the formation of α-ketonic acid, decarboxylation and generation of CO_2. Through these activities, Vitamin B1 benefits the prevention and treatment of sugar metabolic

| Drinking tea frequently is beneficial for diabetes, and most of the ways of making tea are simple and convenient.

disturbance. As a coenzyme, pantothenic acid in tea plays an important part in metabolism of sugar, protein and fat. In addition "6, 8-dylipoic acid" in tea combines with Vitamin B$_1$ into cocarboxylase, which helps prevent sugar metabolic disturbance.

Patients with diabetes can drink green tea therapeutically, and often drinking green tea can also prevent diabetes in normal people. Single tea is effective for preventing and treating diabetes, keeping the following in mind: the effect of green tea is better than that of black tea; the effect of old tea is better than that of new tea; and the effect of cold tea is better than that of hot tea.

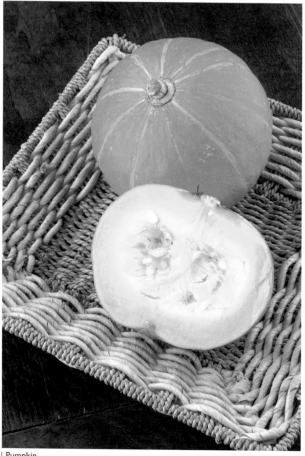

| Pumpkin.

1. Cold tea

Ingredient: 10 g crude tea leaves.

Procedure: Soak the leaves in 200 ml of cold (previously-boiled) water for 5 hours.

Usage: Three times per day, 50–150 ml per time. Persist in taking it for 40–60 days for maximum curative effect.

Efficacy: It is taken to relieve the symptoms of diabetes. Patients with comparatively serious states of illness can keep taking it for a longer period of time.

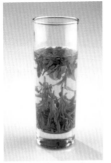

| Green tea leaves in the water.

2. Pumpkin tea

Ingredient: 250 g pumpkin.

Procedure: Cut fresh pumpkin into small pieces, or grind dried pumpkin into rough powder. Decoct the pumpkin pieces or 50 g pumpkin powder with water, get the extraction and put it in a vacuum flask.

Usage: One dose per day. Take it frequently whenever you like.

Efficacy: It reduces blood sugar, lipids and blood pressure. It is mainly taken for diabetes, hypertension and hyperlipidemia.

3. Corn silk green tea

Ingredients: 15 g corn silk, 0.5 g green tea leaves.

Procedure: Put the corn silk in 300 ml of water, boil it for 5 minutes, and then add green tea leaves.

Usage: One to two doses per day. Split into three portions to drink at different times.

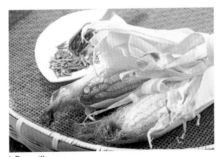

| Corn silk tea.

Efficacy: It is taken by patients with diabetes whose urine is turbid, appearing like grease.

4. Waxgourd and watermelon peel tea

Ingredients: 1,000 g fresh peel of Chinese waxgourd, 1,000 g fresh watermelon peel, 250 g snakegourd fruit, 500 g white sugar.

Procedure: Remove the external layer of the fresh peel of Chinese waxgourd and fresh watermelon peel, and then cut into thin slices.

Mash the snakegourd fruit. Boil these three things together for 1 hour. Get the extraction, and concentrate it over low flame until nearly dry. Add white sugar, mix evenly, and put in a bottle for future use.

Usage: Two to three times per day, and 10 g per time.

Efficacy: It can clear internal heat, promote secretion of saliva or body fluid, and quench thirst. It is mainly taken for diabetes.

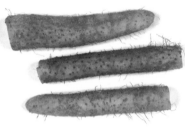

| Chinese yam.

5. Chinese yam tea

Ingredients: 250 g Chinese yam.

Procedure: Decoct with water.

Usage: Drink it as a tea substitute.

Efficacy: It can promote vitality, tonify *yin*, and quench thirst. It is taken for diabetes.

6. Salt ginger tea

Ingredients: 2 slices ginger, 4.5 g salt, 6 g green tea leaves.

Procedure: Simmer for 500 ml of extraction.

Usage: Separate into several portions to take at different times.

Efficacy: It is taken for thirst, polydipsia (thirst with excessive fluid intake), discontentment or restlessness, and copious urine.

7. Water spinach and corn silk tea

Ingredients: 250 g fresh water spinach, 200 g corn silk.

Procedure: Add fresh water to decoct water spinach and corn silk for extraction.

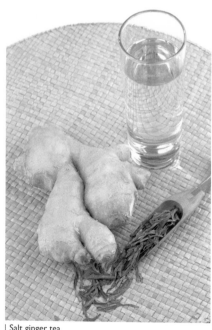

| Salt ginger tea.

Usage: Drink it as a tea substitute. One dose per day.

Efficacy: It has the effects of reducing blood sugar, promoting diuresis, and clearing internal heat and toxic materials. It is mainly taken for:

- diabetes, thirst, polydipsia and copious urine;
- nephropathy, edema and oliguria (low urine output);
- hepatitis and jaundice;
- hematemesis, hemoptysis or hematuria (vomiting, coughing or urinating blood).

8. Prescription of bitter melon

Ingredients: 150 g fresh bitter melon.

Procedure: Cook the fresh bitter melon thoroughly with oil and salt.

Usage: Eat the dish. If dried bitter melon is used, drink it as a tea substitute. Once a day.

Efficacy: It is taken for diabetes.

9. Prescription of black fungus

Ingredients: Black fungus, dolichos seeds.

Procedure: Dry an equal amount of black fungus and dolichos seeds in the sun, and grind them into powder.

Usage: Take 9 g each time with boiled water.

Efficacy: It is taken for diabetes.

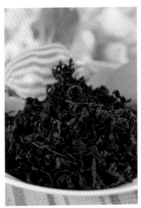

| Black fungus.

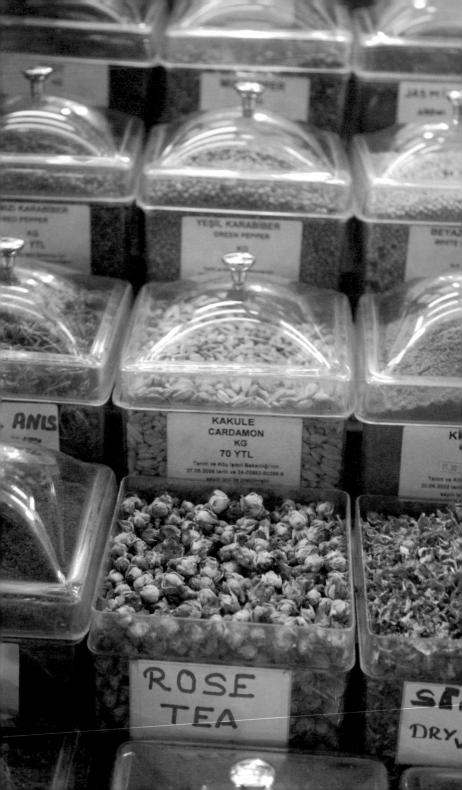

Chapter 12
Anti-aging, Topical Treatments and Other Health Care

There is widespread documentation through the ages of the belief that tea is good for health and longevity. As just one example, in the Qing dynasty classic *Notes Taken at the Lotus Corridor* it is written that tea can "preserve one's health and lengthen one's life." Numerous notable figures, including Qianlong, an emperor in the Qing dynasty, Wu Juenong, who enjoyed the title of "Tea Saint in contemporary times," and Eisai, a Zen master with the title of "Tea Saint in Japan," appreciated tea and promoted its life-prolonging aspect.

| Since tea therapy serves to ease pain from diseases and improve quality of life, it is becoming widely popular.

Aging

The effect of tea in prolonging life is related to its nutritional and pharmacological ingredients, among which tea polyphenols and vitamins A, E and C make the greatest contribution.

As for understanding and preventing aging, there is a theory about the role of "radicals." The human body continually consumes oxygen during the process of breathing, which generates radicals. Aging is caused by excessive radicals in the human body. Radicals are highly reactive, being capable of, directly or indirectly, causing strong oxidation.

Polyphenols in tea can combat radicals, with those in extraction of green tea capable of reaching 98%. Studies in Japan have proven the effect of tea polyphenols in preventing the aging of cells and fighting senility. Vitamin E, commonly used to delay senility, has only a 4% effect in preventing peroxidation of fatty acid, while that of green tea rich in tea polyphenol is as high as 74%.

The peroxidation process of fat greatly harms human health, for example causing anemia, arteriosclerosis and diabetes. Vitamin C and Vitamin E in tea are of very strong anti-oxidant activity.

In addition multi-amino acids in tea are also effective in anti-aging. Cystine can promote hair growth, and prevent and treat premature senility. Lysine, threonine, and histidine can enhance growth and intellectual development, increase the absorption of calcium and iron, and prevent senile osteoporosis and anemia. The microelement fluorine can also prevent senile osteoporosis. Of course, as stated in other chapters of this book, tea can prevent and treat many other diseases, which is also important for prolonging life.

The effect of tea in prevent aging can be realized with single prescription of tea irrespective of variety. Therefore, a regular practice of drinking tea is important in the fight against growing old. The type of tea you take may reflect the season. In spring, people can take scented tea with strong aroma, because the aroma has a strong releasing effect, ridding the body of cold-evil accumulated in the winter and enabling *yang qi* to gradually ascend and emit. Summer is the best season to drink green tea. The nature of green tea is cold and bitter, so it is the most appropriate to drink it in summer.

For autumn and winter, oolong and black tea, respectively, are recommended. The nature of oolong tea is between those of black tea and green tea, and it has properties of both, being suitable for a transitional season. If there is no oolong tea, it is acceptable to mix black and green tea so that the effects of the two can both be realized, and the taste is quite unique. In winter, it is proper to drink black tea that is sweet in taste and warm in nature, being capable of harmonizing the stomach and nourishing the liver as well as helping to enhance *yang qi*. These qualities also make black tea especially appropriate for the elderly.

1. Baxian tea

Ingredients: 750 g rice, 750 g millet, 750 g soy beans, 750 g azuki beans (small red bean), 750 g mung beans, 500 g tea leaves, 375 g black sesame, 75 g flower pepper, 150 g fennel, 30 g dried ginger, 30 g fried crystal salt.

Procedure: Fry the first five ingredients until fragrant. Then grind all these ingredients

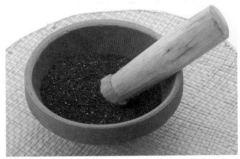

| Black sesame.

into a fine powder, and fry the powder till it becomes yellow. Add a few walnuts, jujubes, pine nuts and white sugar, and store in a porcelain jar.

Usage: Three times per day, and 6–9 g per time, infused with boiling water.

Efficacy: It has the effects of tonifying the spirit and lifting one's mood, promoting vitality, and tonifying the kidneys. It is taken for anti-aging, poor health and malnutrition.

2. Pearl tea

Ingredients: Pearls, tea leaves.

Procedure: Grind the pearl into extremely fine powder.

Usage: Take 2–3 g pearl powder with tea. Once every 10 days.

Efficacy: It can moisten the skin, preserve youth and beautify the appearance. It is effective for aging of facial skin, diseases and overall aging.

3. Chinese cornbind and pine tea

Ingredients: 18 g Chinese cornbind, 30 g pine needle (pine flower is preferred if available), 5 g oolong tea leaves.

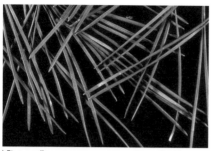

| Pine needle.

Procedure: First decoct Chinese cornbind and pine needle or flower with water for about 20 minutes, and then use the extraction to make oolong tea.

Usage: Take it whenever you like.

Efficacy: It has the effects of tonifying the spirit and replenishing blood, and strengthening the body's immunity to eliminate pathogenic factors. It is beneficial for those with deficiency of liver-*yin* and kidney-*yin*, people engaged in chemical/radioactive or underground mining work as well as patients with leucopenia (decreased white blood cells) after chemoradiotherapy.

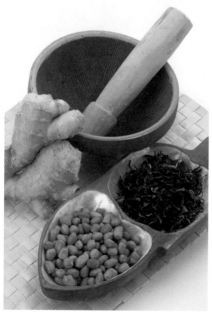

| Ground peanut ginger tea.

4. Ground peanut ginger tea

Ingredients: Tea leaves, peanuts, ginger.

Procedure: Grind these in a bowl or with mortar and pestle.

Usage: Drink it, infused with boiling water.

Efficacy: It helps to prevent diseases and aging, protect health and prolong life.

5. Rhubarb tea

Ingredients: 6 g green tea leaves, 2 g rhubarb.

Procedure: Infuse with boiling water.

Usage: Drink it whenever you feel thirsty.

Efficacy: It has the effects of clearing internal heat, purging intense internal heat, relaxing the bowels, removing food retention and alleviating flatulency. Drinking this tea often can delay aging.

Fatigue

In modern society, fatigue is a major danger to health. If people experience physiological fatigue for a long time, they will eventually break down from constant overwork and come to a state of pathological fatigue, bringing harm to the immune system. This is reflected in the saying relating to the body's energy: "If there is vital *qi* inside the human body, the evil *qi* cannot invade. If there is evil *qi* inside the body, the vital *qi* will inevitably become weak."

As a result, adopting such measures as making sure to combine rest with exertion, having a reasonable diet, maintaining a positive outlook, ensuring adequate sleep and taking proper exercises is very necessary. Another effective way to combat fatigue and preserve one's health is through tea therapy.

To eliminate ordinary fatigue, people need only take single tea. If people experience fatigue over a long period, or have a fatigue syndrome, they can adopt the complex prescription of tea therapy, using herbs together with tea to recuperate.

The effect of tea in stimulating the nervous system can bring high spirits and promote mental activity. In terms of the motor system, tea can also relieve fatigue. On the one hand, caffeine in tea helps enable calcium ions to be discharged to enhance skeletal muscle contraction, and on the other, it neutralizes the acidoids in muscles to strengthen them and allay tiredness.

1. Honey lemon tea

Ingredients: Tea leaves, half a lemon, two spoonfuls of honey.

Procedure: Decoct tea leaves for a spoonful of strong extraction. Wash the lemon and extract juice. Then pour the juice into a cup with prepared tea. Mix together and add some honey.

Usage: Add boiling water and drink.

Efficacy: It can allay fatigue.

2. Lotus seed rock candy tea

Ingredients: 5 g tea leaves, 30 g lotus seeds, 20 g rock candy.

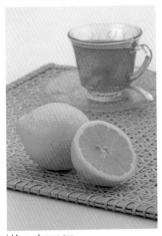

| Honey lemon tea.

Procedure: First soak lotus seeds in warm water for several hours. Then stew seeds with rock candy and water until mushy. Simmer tea leaves in boiling water. Take the extraction and combine it with the lotus seed mixture.

Usage: One dose per day. Take it whenever you like.

Efficacy: It has the effects of relieving mental strain and strengthening the kidneys, clearing internal heat in the heart and calming the mind. It is taken for deficient heart *qi*, palpitation, and related conditions.

3. Five-leaf gynostemma green tea

Ingredients: 15 g herb of five-leaf gynostemma, 2 g green tea leaves.

Procedure: First, roast or bake the five-leaf gynostemma to get rid of fishy smell. Grind it into powder and soak it with tea leaves in boiling water for 10 minutes. Or decoct these two things with water for 10 minutes.

Usage: One dose per day. Take it whenever you like. You may add honey or white sugar to taste.

Efficacy: It has the effects of tonifying the five internal organs and strengthening the physique. It is taken for asthenic syndromes, especially for chronic ailment or weakness, insomnia, hepatitis B, ulcer, tuberculosis, chronic tracheitis (inflammation of the trachea), heart disease, hypertension and hyperlipidemia.

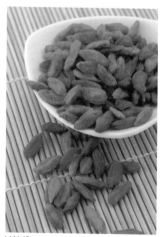

| Wolfberry.

4. Strength-enhancing tea

Ingredients: 3 g tea leaves, 15 g root of manyprickle acanthopanax, 10 g herb of hairyvien agrimonia, 7 g wolfberries.

Procedure: Cut up the root of manyprickle acanthopanax, and simmer it with other three ingredients.

Usage: Drink it daily, taking one dose.

Efficacy: It has the effects of tonifying *qi* and enhancing strength, tonifying kidneys and bones, and preventing fatigue.

5. Honey green tea

Ingredients: 5 g green tea leaves,

25 g honey.

Procedure: Put these into a cup, add 300–500 ml of boiling water and soak for 5 minutes.

Usage: Take it when it is warm, or decoct for tea extraction and then add some honey to taste.

Efficacy: It refreshes, tonifies deficiency, and allays tiredness.

6. Pilose asiabell and jujube tea

Ingredients: 3 g tea leaves, 20 g root of pilose asiabell, 15 jujubes.

Procedure: Decoct with water.

Usage: Divide into 2-3 portions, and take one portion daily.

Efficacy: It has the effects of tonifying the spleen, harmonizing the stomach, supplementing *qi* and promoting the production of body fluid. It is appropriate for people with dry eyes due to chronic fatigue syndrome.

7. Chrysanthemum green tea

Ingredients: 3 g green tea leaves (longjing tea is the best), 10 g chrysanthemum.

Procedure: Infuse with boiling water and cover it for a while.

Usage: Drink it as a tea substitute.

Efficacy: It has the effects of removing internal heat in the liver, improving eyesight, dispelling wind and relieving pain. It is appropriate for people who have blurred vision or headache due to chronic fatigue syndrome.

8. Szechwan lovage tea

Ingredients: 6 g green tea leaves, 6 g rhizome of Szechwan lovage, brown sugar.

Procedure: Decoct with one and a half cups of water till there is only one cup of extraction.

Usage: Drink it as a tea substitute.

Efficacy: It has the effects of tonifying *qi* and invigorating blood circulation, dispelling wind and relieving pain. It is taken by those suffering from chronic fatigue syndrome with headache and blood deficiency.

9. Hairyvien agrimonia and jujube tea

Ingredients: 45 g herb of hairyvien agrimonia, 30 g jujubes.

Procedure: Decoct with water for half an hour.

Usage: Drink it frequently as a tea substitute. One dose per day.

Efficacy: It has the effects of strengthening the body's resistance, tonifying deficiency and strengthening muscles. It is taken for body weakness, low spirits and lassitude.

Radiation Damage

Radiation damage can cause a variety of functional disorders. Due to the comprehensive effect of various ingredients in tea, it can alleviate or get rid of many physiological problems caused by radiation damage. Different kinds of tea have a certain degree of anti-radiation effect.

The first and foremost effective ingredients are tea polyphenols and lipopolysaccharides, which have the desirable property of radiation-resistance. Moreover tea polyphenols can lower the oxygen concentration in tissues to decrease oxidation and weaken the effect of exposure to ionizing radiation. Tea polyphenols can also enhance the vascular wall, and reduce or prevent radiation harm. Lipopolysaccharides can improve non-specific immune function, prevent radiation damage, improve hematopoietic function (production of blood cells) and keep the levels of many components of the blood in balance.

The effect of tea in replenishing the blood is mainly demonstrated by increased white blood cells. Since tea can prevent radiation damage and raise the white blood cell count, it is of vital importance for patients who receive radiotherapy for tumors. It can relieve some side effects of radiotherapy and lower the extent to which white blood cells decrease.

In addition, other components in tea, such as Vitamin C, Vitamin E and caffeine, also have auxiliary pharmacodynamical effects. Tea not only contains rich iron (regular tea-drinkers can obtain one-quarter of the daily requirement for iron from tea) but also Vitamin C, which can promote the absorption of iron. This means that drinking tea can prevent iron-deficiency anemia. Microelements in tea (e.g. copper, and zinc, etc.) can also prevent anemia, while folic acid can prevent megaloblastic anemia.

The effects of tea in replenishing blood and increasing white blood cell counts are obvious. Vitamin C in tea can promote the absorption of iron in diet. However, it has also been found through experiments that some components in tea, together with iron, will form insoluble compounds inside the digestive tract, hence inhibiting the absorption of iron.

Therefore while tea can play a role in preventing anemia, it can be harmful for patients who have anemia. For all those with iron-deficiency anemia and those who are prone to have iron-deficiency anemia due to certain conditions, e.g. pregnant or nursing women, fertile women with menorrhagia, youngsters, babies and children, it is better to drink less tea.

1. Jujube tea
Ingredients: 5 g tea leaves, 10 jujubes, 10 g white sugar.
Procedure: Simmer tea leaves in boiled water and get the extraction. Mix jujubes with white sugar and boil them together in water till the jujubes become mushy. Pour into tea extraction.
Usage: Mix the mushy jujubes and tea evenly.
Efficacy: It has the effects of replenishing blood, tonifying the spirit, strengthening the spleen and harmonizing the stomach. It is taken for anemia, and can also prevent vitamin deficiency.

2. Danshen root and Solomon's seal tea
Ingredients: 5 g tea leaves, 10 g root of danshen, 10 g rhizome of Solomon's seal.
Procedure: Grind into rough powder, infuse with boiling water, and cover for 10 minutes.
Usage: Drink one dose per day.
Efficacy: It invigorates blood circulation, and replenishes blood and energy. It is taken for anemia and to increase white blood cell count.

3. Nourishing sesame tea
Ingredients: 6 g black sesame, 3 g tea leaves.
Procedure: Fry the black sesame till it becomes yellow. Then add tea leaves and decoct with water, or soak the tea and sesame in boiling water and cover for 10 minutes.
Usage: One to two doses per day. Drink the liquid and eat the black sesame and tea leaves.
Efficacy: It has the effects of nourishing the liver and kidneys, nourishing blood and moistening lungs. It is taken to combat deficiency of liver and kidneys, rough skin, dry or premature grey hair, and tinnitus.

4. Wolfberry and schisandra berry tea
Ingredients: Equal amounts of wolfberries and schisandra berries.

Procedure: Grind into powder, and infuse with boiling water.

Usage: Twice per day, 5 g per time. Drink it as a tea substitute, eating the solids.

Efficacy: It nourishes human essence and blood, and is taken to remedy deficiencies of these two things, as well as dizziness, tinnitus, palpitation, insomnia, blurred vision, spermatorrhea and chronic hepatitis.

Summer Heat

Whenever it is summer, with strong sunshine and high temperatures, people often feel sweaty, thirsty, dizzy and weak. At this time, a cup of green tea is recommended.

As for why drinking tea can slake thirst, there are many reasons if analyzing from the perspective of science. First of all, the feeling of thirst results from water deficiency inside the cells, and drinking tea is a good way to replenish the water. In addition, after combining with various aromatic substances, tea polyphenols can slightly stimulate oral mucous membranes, helping to promote salivary secretion, keep the mouth moist, and relieve thirst.

Sweating can reduce such components as sodium, calcium, potassium, Vitamin B and Vitamin C in the body, hence increasing the sense of thirst. Tea is rich in Vitamin C, which promotes the absorption of oxygen in cells, alleviates the reaction to heat, and increases salivary secretion. The potassium in tea can reach as high as 1.5%–2.5%, which helps replenish the potassium lost through sweating.

Other components help regulate body temperature. It has been reported that tea can promote sweat gland secretion, enabling moisture to evaporate from the skin and dissipate heat. Caffeine can help control the brain's thermoregulation center from the inside to reduce summer heat. Moreover, caffeine, theophylline and theobromine in tea can promote diuresis, removing heat to decrease body temperature, thus relieving summer heat.

Therefore, tea is an ideal drink to prevent heatstroke, quench thirst and promote the secretion of saliva or body fluids.

1. Salt tea
Ingredients: Tea leaves, salt.

Procedure: Brew with boiling water.

Usage: Take it directly.

Efficacy: It has the effects of clearing internal heat, relieving summer heat, replenishing body fluid and quenching thirst.

2. Jasmine combination tea

Ingredients: 3 g jasmine, 3 g oolong tea leaves, 6 g wrinkled gianthyssop, 6 g lotus leaves (chopped up into thin strips).

Procedure: Soak in boiling water for 5–10 minutes.

Usage: 1–2 doses per day. Take it frequently whenever you like.

Efficacy: It can clear summer heat and resolve dampness. It is taken for the feeling of summer heat and dampness in summer, fever and fullness in the head, a sense of suppression in the chest, lack of appetite, and infrequent or insufficient urine.

3. Mixed berry tea for summer

Ingredients: Equal amounts of wolfberries and schisandra berries.

Procedure: Grind into powder, infuse with boiling water. Seal, and wait for 3 days before taking.

Usage: Drink it as a tea substitute whenever you like, every day.

Efficacy: It has the effects of clearing summer heat, relieving fatigue and replenishing vital essence. It is mainly taken for summer non-acclimation, excessive sweating due to physical labor, deficiency of *yin*, thirst, deficiency syndrome of lungs, and cough.

4. Bitter melon tea

Ingredients: One bitter melon, green tea leaves.

Procedure: Cut open the upper end of a fresh bitter melon, get rid of the pulp, and put the green tea leaves into it. Hang the melon in a place with good ventilation. After drying it in shade, wash the outside and wipe dry. Then cut it up (together with the tea leaves), mix thoroughly, and put in a vacuum flask. Infuse with boiling water, cover tightly and soak for half an hour.

Usage: 10 g per time. Drink it frequently.

Efficacy: It cures heatstroke and fever, excessive or abnormal thirst, and difficult

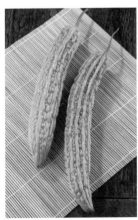

| Bitter melon.

urination.

5. Old tea leaf therapy
Ingredient: 15 g old tea leaves.
Procedure: Infuse with hot water.
Usage: Drink it whenever you feel thirsty. Take it often.
Efficacy: It has the effects of clearing internal heat, excreting sputum and relieving pain.

Toxic Heat

The word "toxin" has a wide range of meanings. Tea is effective against toxins caused by disease (e.g. some inflammations and infections) as well as some diseases caused by toxins. According to TCM theory, most toxins are classified as "hot" so tea works by dissipating internal heat to detoxify.

The development of modern industry has brought prosperity and other advantages but has also caused environmental pollution. When the contents of various heavy metals (copper, lead, mercury and chromium, for example) are too high in food and potable water, it can be toxic to human health.

As proven by many experiments, when polyphenol in tea mixes with heavy metals, it forms a precipitate, which is insoluble. Since these insoluble substances cannot be absorbed by the intestines, they will not cause harm to the body.

We have seen before that tea has a diuresis-promoting essence. When it encounters some poisonous metals, such as aluminum, zinc, stibium and mercury, which have invaded the body, a chemical reaction will occur, making a soluble substance. This can be discharged with urine, hence having the effect of detoxification. Tea can not only precipitate cadmium, but also contains zinc, which is an antagonist of cadmium. Therefore, drinking tea can eliminate the harm of cadmium.

The effect of detoxification of some drugs is realized by caffeine in tea. Caffeine can stimulate the nervous system, antagonizing the doping effect. Furthermore caffeine can improve the metabolic capacity (including the function of detoxification) of the liver, enhance the circulation of blood, and accelerate the discharge of drugs out of blood.

Smoking harms human health in many ways. After getting into the body, the nicotine from a cigarette increases hormone secretion to promote vasoconstriction, which affects blood circulation, decreases the oxygen supply and causes blood pressure to rise. Smoking can also accelerate arteriosclerosis, reduce Vitamin C in the body and accelerate aging. As we have seen, tea contains comparatively high levels of Vitamin C, many substances that strengthen vessels, and ingredients that restrain such carcinogenic substances as benzopyrene and aflatoxin. Moreover catechin in tea can discharge hazardous substances out of the body. Smokers who drink tea can relieve some toxic actions of cigarettes, but only to a certain extent.

1. Honeysuckle flower tea
Ingredient: 500 g honeysuckle.
Procedure: Add 1,000 ml of water and soak for 2 hours.
Usage: Drink it as a tea substitute. Twice per day, 50 ml per time.
Efficacy: It can prevent and treat heat rash.

2. Dandelion tea
Ingredients: 30 g fresh dandelion or 20 g dried dandelion.
Procedure: Add water, and take the extraction as tea.
Usage: One dose per day. Frequently take it whenever you like.
Efficacy: It can treat heat rash and acute suppurative infection caused by summer heat.

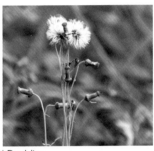
| Dandelion.

3. Detoxifying chrysanthemum tea
Ingredients: 2 g tea leaves, 2 g chrysanthemum.
Procedure: Infuse with boiling water for 6 minutes.
Usage: Take one cup after each meal every day.
Efficacy: It has the effects of removing heat, detoxifying, clearing the liver, improving vision, relieving cough, stopping pain, lowering lipid levels and preventing aging.

Bacterial Infection and Inflammation

Bacteriostasis refers to inhibiting the growth of pathogenic bacteria and other microorganisms. Diminishing inflammation is the alleviation or elimination of lesions or other manifestations caused by bacteria or other reasons. According to Bergey's Manual of Systematic Bacteriology, there are altogether nineteen class groups of bacteria, and tea polyphenol and its derivatives can inhibit the activity of nearly 100 kinds of bacteria belonging to twelve of these class groups.

Flavanols in tea help inflammation through hormonal activity. They work in promoting the activity of the adrenal glands, reducing the permeability of blood capillaries, decreasing exudation of blood, and fighting against histamine. Flavanol compounds themselves can also directly diminish inflammation. As a result, there are practices of treating wounds with tea to prevent and treat inflammation.

Catechin compounds in tea can obviously inhibit various pathogenic bacteria like typhoid bacillus, paratyphoid bacillus, yellow hemolytic staphylococcus, golden yellow streptococcus, and shigella dysenteriae. The higher the grade of green tea, the better the effect of inhibiting bacterial activity.

Due to the comprehensive effect of many components in tea, as well as the way it can protect against hazardous substances, most of the pathogenic bacteria (as well as viruses) can be inhibited, and organs protected and purified.

1. Corktree and cocklebur tea

Ingredients: 9 g bark of Chinese corktree, 10 g fruit of Siberian cocklebur, 3 g green tea leaves.

Procedure: Grind into rough powder and infuse with boiling water for 10 minutes, or simmer for extraction.

Usage: One dose per day, separated into two portions to take at different times.

Efficacy: It has the effects of clearing internal heat, dispersing blood stasis, removing discharge, detoxifying, and improving hearing through clearing ear infection (otitis media).

2. Detoxifying wild chrysanthemum tea

Ingredients: 25 g wild chrysanthemum.

Procedure: Put the wild chrysanthemum in a vacuum flask, infuse with boiling water, and cover for 15 minutes. 5 g of licorice root may be added (optional).

Usage: Take it frequently as a tea substitute. One dose per day. It can also be used externally by simmering wild chrysanthemum, and using the extraction to wash the affected area, 3–4 times per day.

Efficacy: It has the effects of detoxifying, clearing internal heat and relieving swelling and pain. It is mainly taken for summer heat and inflammation of the hair follicle. It tastes bitter and can easily impair stomach *qi*, so it mustn't be taken by people with deficiency of stomach *qi*.

3. Mung bean and licorice tea

Ingredients: 60 g mung beans, 15 g licorice root.

Procedure: Grind the beans and licorice into rough powder. Put into a vacuum flask and infuse with boiling water. Cover for 20 to 30 minutes.

Usage: Drink it frequently as a tea substitute. Take one dose in the daytime and one dose at night. When necessary, you may take one dose every 6 hours.

Efficacy: It has the effects of clearing heat and detoxifying.

Skin and Hair Problems

We now understand that the health and beauty of the skin and hair is mainly related to the intake of various nutrients. For example, the lack of Vitamin A can easily lead to dry and rough skin and affect the production of hair and nails. Insufficient Vitamin B_2 can cause inflammation of the skin of the lips and seborrheic dermatitis. The lack of Vitamin B_5 will result in pellagra, and when exposed to sunlight, skin will become red and swollen, painful and itchy, and rough. If one does not have enough Vitamin C, the fragility of the vessels will increase and petechial hemorrhages can take place. The lack of Vitamin E can easily cause skin pigmentation. Finally, insufficient proteins and necessary fatty acids will also make skin rough, ashy or dull without luster, and appear old.

Tea contains abundant Vitamin C, Vitamin E and other nutrients that can replenish deficiencies in the human body. Moreover, polyphenols (especially catechin) in tea can inhibit bacteria, diminish inflammation, prevent oxidation, prevent the formation of lipofuscin, and absorb toxins such as melanin and discharge them out of body. Chlorogenic acid in tea can also protect skin. Therefore, tea, both for internal and external use, has a definite beautifying effect.

1. Milk black tea
Ingredients: 3 g black tea leaves, 100 g milk, salt.
Procedure: First simmer black tea leaves for strong extraction. Boil the milk and put in a cup. Pour the black tea extraction into the milk, add some salt and mix.
Usage: Drink it as a tea substitute.
Efficacy: It has the effects of moistening the skin, preserving youth and beauty, and strengthening the physique, which helps to tonify *qi* and build additional strength.

2. Black sesame tea
Ingredients: Black tea leaves, black sesame.
Procedure: Mix black tea leaves and black sesame, then grind them into powder.
Usage: Eat half a small spoonful of the powder each time. Twice per day, once in the morning and once in the afternoon.
Efficacy: It has the effects of moistening the five internal organs, improving eyesight, and darkening the beard and hair. It is especially suitable for people with weakness, premature grey hair, anemia, dry and rough skin, dizziness and tinnitus, and dry stool or constipation.

3. Lingzhi mushroom green tea
Ingredients: 10 g lingzhi mushroom, a small amount of green tea leaves.
Procedure: Cut lingzhi mushroom into thin slices, infuse with boiling water, and add green tea leaves.
Usage: Drink it as a tea substitute.
Efficacy: It not only tonifies middle *jiao* and *qi*, but also reinforces muscles and bones. It helps keep one's spirit young and skin white and soft.

4. Chinese cornbind combination tea
Ingredients: An equal amount of green tea leaves, Chinese cornbind, rhizome of oriental water plantain and root of danshen.
Procedure: Decoct with water and get the extraction.
Usage: Drink one dose per day. You may divide into portions to drink at separate times as you wish.
Efficacy: It has the effects of beautifying the face and hair, lowering lipid levels and reducing weight.

Appendices

Bibliography

Ancient Medical Books

bencao gangmu [Compendium of Materia Medica] by Li Shizhen, Ming dynasty

bencao shiyi [Gleaning Herbs] by Chen Cangqi, Tang dynasty

binhu jijianfang [Bin Hu Collection of Simple Prescriptions] by Li Shizhen, Ming dynasty

hanshi yitong [Han's Book on Medicine] by Han Mao, Song dynasty

huangdi neijing [Yellow Emperor's Inner Canon], Warring States

guang ya [Guangya] by Zhangyi, Wei dynasty

heji jufang [Prescriptions of Peaceful Benevolent Dispensary], Song dynasty

jiayong liangfang [Home Remedy] edited by Gong Zizhang, Ming dynasty

jinkui yaolue [Synopsis of Golden Chamber] by Zhang Zhongjing, Han dynasty

puji fang [Prescriptions for Universal Relief] by Zhu Di, etc., Ming dynasty

qianjin fang [Prescriptions Worth a Thousand in Gold] by Sun Simiao, Tang dynasty

qianjin yifang [Supplement to Essential Prescriptions Worth a Thousand Gold] by Sun Simiao, Tang dynasty

shanghan zabing lun [Treatise on Febrile and Miscellaneous Diseases] by Zhang Zhongjing, Han dynasty

shesheng zhongmiaofang [Various Nostrums for Conserving One's Health] by Zhang Shiche, Ming dynasty

shengji zonglu [General Records of Holy Universal Relief] edited by Zhao Ji, etc., Song dynasty

shijian bencao [Food Reference to Materia Medica] by Fei Boxiong, Qing dyansty

shiliao bencao [Dietary Therapy of Materia Medica] by Meng Shen, Tang dynasty

shiyi dexiaofang [Effective Formulas Proved by Physicians for Generations] by Wei Yilin, Yuan dynasty *taiping shenghuifang* [Peaceful Holy Benevolent Prescriptions] by Wang Huaiyin, Song dynasty

waitai miyao [Medical Secrets of an Official] by Wang Tao, Tang dynasty

xinxiu bencao [Tang Materia Medica] collectively complied by Su Jing and others, Tang dynasty

yibu quanlu [Whole Records of Medical Books] edited by Chen Menglong, Qing dynasty

yinshan zhengyao [Principles of Correct Diet] by Hu Sihui, Yuan dynasty

Modern and Contemporary Medical Books

Chen Keji, *cixi guangxu yifang xuanyi* [Imperial Medicaments—Medical Prescriptions Written for Empress Dowager Cixi and Emperor Guangxu with Commentary]. Beijing: zhonghua shuju (Zhonghua Book Company), 1981.

Chen Zongmao, *zhongguo chajing* [Chinese Classic of Tea]. Shanghai: Shanghai wenhua chubanshe (Shanghai Cultural Press), 1992.

Cheng Li, *chajiu zhi baibing* [Various Kinds of Diseases Cured by Tea and Wine]. Shanghai: Shanghai kexue jishu wenxian chubanshe (Shanghai Science and Technology Literature Press), 1991.

China Food Periodical Office, *chaye shiyong zhishi* [Practical Knowledge about Tea]. Beijing: guoji wenhua chubanshe gongsi (International Cultural Publishing Company), 1988.

Chinese Food Periodical Office, *yinshi liaofa 100 li* [100 Cases of Diet Therapy]. Beijing: zhongguo shipin chubanshe (Chinese Food Press), 1985.

Dang Yi, *yincha yu yangsheng 400 wen* [400 Questions about Tea-Drinking and Health-Care]. Beijing: zhongguo yixue keji chubanshe (Chinese Medical Science and Technology Press), 1995.

Former Revolutionary Committee of the Academy of Traditional Chinese Medicine, *changjianbing yanfang yanjiu cankao ziliao* [Reference Material for Research on Proved Recipes of Common Diseases]. Beijing: renmin weisheng chubanshe (People's Medical Publishing House), 1970.

Former Revolutionary Committee of the Institute of Traditional Chinese Medicine in Changchun, *Jilin zhongcaoyao* [Chinese Medicinal Herbs in Jilin Province]. Changchun: Jilin renmin chubanshe (Jilin People's Publishing

House), 1970.

Hu Haitian and Liang Jianhui, *yinshi yu liaofa* [Diet and Therapy]. Guangzhou: Guangdong keji chubanshe (Guangdong Science and Technology Press), 1981.

Hu Ximing, *zhongguo zhongyi mifang daquan* [Secret Prescription of Traditional Chinese Medicine in China]. Shanghai: wenhui chubanshe (Wenhui Press), 1989.

Huang Rongzong, *jinan zhongzheng xinfangjie* [New Prescriptions for Acute, Difficult and Serious Illnesses]. Fuzhou: Fujian kexue jishu chubanshe (Fujian Science and Technology Press), 1989.

Institute of Pharmaceutics in Fujian Province, *Fujian zhongcaoyao* [Chinese Medicinal Herbs in Fujian Province]. Fujian: Fujian yiyao gongsi (Fujian Medical Corporation), 1970.

Jin Guoliang, *yangsheng zhibing chaliao fang* [Prescriptions of Tea Therapy for Health-Care and Disease-Treatment]. Shanghai: Shanghai kexue jishu chubanshe (Shanghai Science and Technology Press), 1991.

Lin Qianliang, *yangsheng chashou* [Health-Care and Tea-Related Longevity]. Hong Kong: xianggang jinhui chubanshe (Hong Kong Jinhui Press), 1984.

Liu Qiang, *cha de baojian gongneng yu yaoyong bianfang* [Healthcare Applications and Therapeutic Recipes of Tea]. Beijing: Beijing jindun chubanshe (Beijing Jindun Press), 1990.

Mao Xiao, *zhongguo yaocha* [Chinese Herb Tea]. Shanghai: Shanghai keji chubanshe (Shanghai Science and Technology Press), 1991.

Miao Zhenglai, *zhongyi liangyao liangfang* [Effective Medicine and Prescriptions of Traditional Chinese Medicine]. Beijing: zhongguo yiyao keji chubanshe (Medical Science and Technology Press of China), 1991.

Pang Guoming and Xu Liuguo, *jiating qiaoyong chajiu zhi baibing* [Skillful Use of Tea and Wine for Treating Various Illnesses at Home]. Beijing: zhongguo zhongyiyao chubanshe (Traditional Medicine Press of China), 1991.

pianfang daquan [Folk Prescriptions]. Beijing: Beijing kexue jishu chubanshe (Beijing Science and Technology Press), 1987.

Shang Dejun, *shiyong zhongyi waikexue* [Practical Surgery of Chinese Medicine]. Jinan: Shandong kexue jishu chubanshe (Shandong Science and Technology Press), 1986.

Sichuan zhongyao zhi [Chinese Medicinal Herbs in Sichuan]. Chengdu: Sichuan renmin chubanshe (Sichuan People's Publishing House), 1978.

Tea Science Society of China and Chinese Tea Import and Export Corporation, *zhongguocha yu jiankang* [Chinese Tea and Health]. Beijing: zhongguo duiwai jingji maoyi chubanshe (International Business and Economics Press of China), 1990.

Wang Fuchun and Liu Yang, *yaocha zhi baibing* [Various Illnesses Cured by Herb Tea]. Changchun: Jilin kexue jishu chubanshe (Jilin Science and Technology Press), 1993.

Wang Zhen, *shiwu liaofa jingcui* [Succinct Diet Therapy]. Taiyuan: Shanxi Science and Education Press, 1985.

Xie Guan, *zhongguo yixue dacidian* [Grand Dictionary of Chinese Medicine]. Beijing: zhongguo zhongyiyao chubanshe (China Traditional Chinese Medicine Press), 1994.

Xie Yongxin, *baibing yinshi ziliao* [Autotherapy of Various Diseases through Diet Therapy]. Beijing: zhongyi guji chubanshe (Chinese Medical Book Press), 1987.

Yang Sipeng, *baibing zhongyi yaocha liaofa* [Herb Tea Therapy of Traditional Chinese Medicine for Various Diseases]. Beijing: xueyuan chubanshe (Academy Press), 1994.

Ye Xianchun, *changyong fangji shouce* [Handbook for Common Prescriptions]. Shanghai: Shanghai kexue jishu chubanshe (Shanghai Science and Technology Press), 1958.

Zhang Zheyong and Chen Jinlin, *zhongguo chajiu cidian* [Tea and Wine Dictionary of China]. Changsha: Hunan chubanshe (Hunan Press), 1992.

Index